D0169691

Embracing What Remains

A Memoir

Andrea Couture

Embracing What Remains: A Memoir by Andrea Couture
Published by HJH Press
PO Box 746 Contoocook, New Hampshire 03229

Copyright © 2021 Andrea Couture
All rights reserved. No portion of this book may be reproduced in any form without permission from the publisher, except as permitted by U.S. copyright law. For permissions contact: andreacouture.author@gmail.com.

Cover by Jade Rawlings
Editor: Danielle Anderson, Ink Worthy Books
ISBN: 978-0-578-92826-5 (paperback)
Printed in the United States of America
First Edition

Disclaimer:

The information shared in this book is designed to document the author's personal story on the subjects discussed. This book is not meant to be used, nor should it be used, to diagnose or treat any medical condition. The author is not a medical doctor. For diagnosis or treatment of any medical problem, consult your own physician. The publisher and author are not responsible for any specific health needs that may require medical supervision and are not liable for any damages or negative consequences from any treatment, action, application or preparation, to any person reading or following the information in this book. Some names have been changed to protect privacy. The author has retold her story to the best of her memory and ability to convey the truth as it occurred.

For Dad

1

———◆—◆—◆———

I had to assume the sink was his destination, as my father got up from the table after he finished lunch. He did not answer me when I asked where he was headed. A man on a mission, he kept moving across the honey-colored oak floor in his slippers that made a whispered shush as he shuffled. My father went to perform a task he had done thousands of times, maybe even a million, over a forty-year career as a surgeon. *He can do it*, I thought. He stopped at the sink and looked down, then up and out the window. The ground was blanketed in a crusty, frozen sheet, and the trees bent and bowed under the weight of the snow as if to honor their onlooker. The trees did not move, and all remained still outside. The mountain had not brought its usually notorious wind with it that day. My father's hands reached out into the black abyss of the sink, but that is where the action ceased.

"Dad, here. Put your hands under the water like this. Look at my hands. See? Dad? Dad? Look at my hands," I said, while I stared at his unmoving hands.

My father and I stood side by side at the kitchen sink in the dream house my parents built only a decade ago. Our heights had caught up, as he aged and shrunk with each passing year. I studied my father's face, as he stared straight ahead out the window, his brown eyes glazed over and unfocused behind his glasses. *He can't do it,* I realized. I finally grabbed his hands, placed them under the faucet, and added soap.

"Dad, can you rub your hands together? Dad? Can you rub your hands together like this?" I asked with more urgency to my voice. He started to rub his thumb and forefinger together on one hand as if he was snapping them.

My father's seventieth birthday had recently passed, and I was showing him how to wash his hands, just as I showed my three-year-old son, Henry. Realizing that made me wilt a little inside. He wasn't really following me. I felt my eyes blur with tears, and a twinge of impatience and annoyance pinched my throat. I knew he was slipping deeper; I knew his disease was eating away more of him. I wanted him to do it on his own. I reached for the dishtowel on the counter and dried his hands. For a moment, I pretended he was a surgeon again and I was his operating room nurse, prepping him for surgery. Maybe this act comforted him, or maybe it confused him. I half joked, "Doctor, your towel." I used this moment of levity to escape the dark reality we were navigating, and for one brief instant, I imagined the man he was five years ago.

***

I glanced out my window as the ground below got smaller and smaller. My left hand grabbed the top of my right hand. I squeezed hard and closed my eyes. I had chosen the window seat over the aisle, as I thought that seeing out the window felt like the lesser of two evils. I decided it didn't really matter where I sat on a plane—I still felt trapped. I hated this part of flying—all of flying, really. They say that the takeoff and landing are always the most dangerous. I said a silent Hail Mary and then I felt the plane level off. The captain's calm voice came over the speaker to welcome us all on the flight from Manchester, New Hampshire, to Chicago O'Hare. I thought that might be one of the last times I traveled to Chicago, as my parents were moving to New Hampshire later that month due to my father's recent announcement to retire. It was time to celebrate the end of an era and welcome a new beginning.

The plane landed safely, and I disembarked alone. My husband, Denis, and my two young children stayed back in New Hampshire; I selfishly wanted to enjoy my father's retirement party without any distractions. I knew it might get emotional, and I wanted to have a glass or three of wine without worrying about putting the kids to bed or chasing them around the next morning. I made the call to the driver to let him know I was ready for pick up. Being alone and in Chicago during the fall transported me back to the nineteen-year-old college student, calling for the same ride home every year that I flew home for holidays. Back then, a bag full of dirty laundry was my only companion. Fifteen years and two kids later, I was barely the same woman, but returning home, it was easy to take on that nostalgic feeling and play the well-worn roles of the middle sister and daughter, rather than mother and wife. That day, the driver didn't deliver me to the suburbs, to the corner house in the neighborhood with the brick laid driveway and through the front door of the home I had spent so many years returning to since graduating high school. Rather, I was going to the hotel down the road where my parents were now living. My parents had placed their house on the market, and it sold three days later, so they decided to live the "suite life."

It was sort of depressing, at first, to think of them living like that, but it turned out my mother enjoyed the quaintness of the room, the daily maid service, and the room service. She still saw her friends regularly and visited her hair stylist and manicurist, but she didn't have the hassle of grocery shopping, and she always had fresh towels. Knowing she was content made me feel better about the fact they were essentially living as tourists in their own town.

My sisters, Amy and Liza, were already at the hotel when I arrived. Amy, the eldest, still lived in Illinois within an hour's drive of my parents, and Liza, my baby sister, made the trip out from Boston. We all gathered around each other and began bantering about clothing, hair, and shoes. The flurry of chatter about the next day's retirement party was muffled, as it was a "surprise" for my dad. My mother had planned a lavish lunch at a mansion that was now owned by the university my father had worked at for the previous twenty-four years. In an attempt to "throw him off the scent," we took him out for lunch. My mother stayed back to relax and have some time to herself before the big festivity the next day. We celebrated with champagne and asked the waitress to take our photo. Just my dad and his three girls... I mean *women*. We were not children anymore. Amy had her career in pharmaceuticals, and Liza was a social worker at a children's hospital. I was a mother of two, and we were all now in our thirties. Life had changed so much since our days of shopping at the outdoor mall and stopping for lunch, as we did that day. My father was ending a career and leaving Illinois, and we three sisters were also bidding farewell to a place that had seen us through our middle school and high school years. Our home in the suburbs of Chicago had been ours during our formative years. Our years of puberty, first dates, dances, bike rides, homework, concerts, sisterly screaming matches about clothes, driver's education, SATs, college applications, braces, and ear piercings were left behind, with only pictures and our memories to remind us. My sisters and I were close, but a span of eight years separated Amy as the oldest and Liza as the youngest, and Amy and I were three and a half years apart. My parents raised us to be independent and trusted us to make the right decisions. They were lenient in allowing us to do things, while still being strict in their expectations. As a parent now, I know this is a tough balance to achieve, but my parents seemed to have mastered it.

One night in high school, I went to a concert with friends. My friend drove, and only after arriving did I realize we were actually in another state. On the way home, our car broke down, and we were stranded, waiting for my friend's father to arrive to pick us up. I called my parents to let them know I would be later than I thought. My father answered the phone without missing a beat, as he always did in the middle of the night as the chief trauma surgeon. He would often need to decide whether the helicopter at the hospital should go out and transport a patient, or he could be called in himself to see a patient. I was nervous for my father's reaction to my news. He had assumed I would be home within the hour, based on where I was *supposed* to have been. When he heard the news of my actual location, his only response was, "Well, I guess you will be getting home when I am leaving for work." He didn't scold me; he didn't get angry. He just made it known, with his tone, that he was disappointed. He often left for work around 6 A.M. every day of the week, so he was right in his prediction when I strolled in around 5:30 that morning. My dad never used many words to get his point across. He really didn't need to. If I could feel his disappointment, it was enough for me to question my actions. I knew I had let him down, and I was ashamed. However, I also knew I was a teenager who made mistakes and had to learn from them. Years later, it became a joke about me going to a concert in Wisconsin. My dad always made sure I knew where I was going before I went.

When I succeeded at something, my dad was proud and rejoiced with me. I wasn't the best student, but if I was able to pull my grades up, my dad was complimentary. He would tell me my hard work had "paid off." He was always willing to help his children achieve their goals, and for a few summers, I worked in his office alongside his team of secretaries. I never really saw him while he worked, but I felt closer to him as I filed papers or used the three-hole punch on documents that he had signed. I would sit outside his office with one of his secretaries but once in a while had to enter his office to return or retrieve something. He was rarely in his office, so whenever I went in there, I wandered a bit. I sat at his desk and spun around in his chair. It was a large corner office with two sides full of half windows that sat four floors above the emergency room. I stood up to look out the window and saw my father's car. It was parked close to the ER door, as he had an assigned parking spot. After all, he was the chairman of surgery and the director of the Shock Trauma Institute. Just past his car was the massive red X on the ground that marked the helicopter landing pad. The office boasted a large enough space for an executive -sized desk, rows of bookshelves filled with medical textbooks and family pictures, a conference table and chairs, a closet that was lined and tightly packed with multiple coats that bared my father's embroidered name and "Department of Surgery," a leather couch, and the best and most impressive part (at least to us kids), a bathroom. This was *the* office to have at the hospital. My father had achieved his goals in life and was sitting, quite literally, at the top.

I was proud to wear my ID badge with the Gamelli name on it when I rode the elevator or went to the cafeteria. When I went to college and was majoring in journalism, he connected me with an internship in the marketing department at the hospital. I knew my father had gotten me the internship, but it was up to me to prove myself. He had provided me with the opportunity and the tools to succeed, but he wouldn't do the work for me. That was what made him a great leader.

Life ending in Illinois was a bittersweet time, but mostly sweet, as I was looking forward to my parents living within a forty-five-minute drive of me in New Hampshire. I was excited to have our relationship grow and flourish as I had always dreamed it might upon him retiring.

The day of the party, our limousine pulled up to the stately mansion. The building was a salmon color with white trim and had beautiful gardens surrounding it. As we rode to lunch that day, I think my father figured out where we were headed and why, but the real surprise for him would be in all those who attended. Some guests had traveled from other states, and my mother had made sure to invite not just colleagues, but also neighbors and even some past patients. I recognized most of the names and faces, but it was very formal as we walked around the mansion rooms and greeted each other. A string quartet played in the library of the mansion, while guests mingled, ate from silver trays of hors d'oeuvres, and sipped drinks. A few times, I was greeted with the line, "Oh, you are one of his daughters, but which one?" and we would begin a conversation. I can't say I blamed anyone, as my sisters and I looked quite a bit alike at that point.

I usually answered with the line, "I'm the middle one, Andrea. I live in New Hampshire and have two kids." Ah, yes, right. The one who had the grandchildren, the famous grandchildren my father raved about to anyone who would listen.

Dr. Gamelli, or as some called him, "Dr. G," sat on a stage set up in the grand entrance of the mansion next to my mother, while guests spoke to him and about him from a podium. If he hadn't been sitting next to them on the stage, the event could have been easily confused as his funeral. We laughed, we cried, we listened to people talk about a man who had changed people's lives, saved them, and led a team of proud and energized people. One story that stood out was from a patient he had treated many years before. The patient was severely burned, and his survival shocked everyone, including my father. He referenced a time my dad visited him on Christmas Day in the hospital. As I heard him speak, I felt ashamed. My face felt hot, as if I was under a spotlight. I stood toward the back of the room, leaning up against the wall, hoping no one would turn and look at me. This must have been the same man he had been treating when I guilted my father one Christmas. He hadn't come home that morning until after ten, and my sisters and I had grown impatient to open our gifts. We felt robbed of our Christmas morning and let my father know it when he eventually walked through the door. He then told us that he visited a patient who was very sick, and it was important he saw him, as he may be the only visitor for him that day. We had not thought much of his comment then, as most young children don't want to hear excuses from their parents. His mid-morning arrival on Christmas was typical of a Saturday for me growing up. Almost every Saturday morning as a child, my cartoon watching ended at 10 A.M. when my father arrived home from a morning of rounds at the hospital. My two sisters and I usually groaned in protest, "Ugh, Dad! We just want to watch TV!" My father didn't come home to relax; he came home to keep us busy. If we even uttered the word "bored," a trash bag full of socks would be placed in front of us. "These all need to be matched! Have fun!" he would say with a smile and a nod. If the weather was decent, he was outside, and we worked alongside him. It was our chance to spend time together, even if it meant stacking wood, raking leaves, or doing other yard work. If I had it my way, we would have played with Barbie's or played "house" with my Cabbage Patch dolls. I knew my only way to spend time with my father was to follow his lead, and I did so as the obedient child I strived to be. If it was summertime and the sun was shining, it was time to wash my dad's car. It was washed, dried, waxed, vacuumed, wiped down, and essentially sterilized on the inside. There were no water fights or soap wars; we were a working crew being led by our chief. His car was basically his operating room on wheels. My father kept his clothes, toiletries, car, work bench, shed, and garage all in neat and perfect order. At times, it felt overwhelming, and at other times, I envied him for it and really appreciated the organization if I needed to find something quickly. Why couldn't I be more like him? Unfortunately, my sisters and I did not inherit these traits, much to his dismay. But he worked on us while we lived under his roof, constantly asking us to pick up our shoes so he didn't trip over them. We'd also hear the occasional shout of, "Whose backpack is this?!?" while he tried to fight his way through the mudroom at night.

My memories continued to flow while the patient detailed his time with my father. I had quick memories—flashes—of my dad just being a dad. I'd think back to the swims in our pool back in the '80s, in our first house where I was born in Vermont. I reminisced about the first time he taught me to ski, when I helped him spread mulch around the trees, and spending Sundays reciting the Our Father at mass, or watching him doze off during the homily. My dad had three modes: work at work, work at home, and relax by working. After 8 P.M., he might have been caught enjoying an episode of *M*A*S*H** or *Star Trek*, but for the most part, my dad's career dictated his entire life. Now as an adult, I like to think I lent my father to the outside world to do better things. To save lives. To make his mark on the medical world and to support his family financially. But, as a child, I assumed his work was more important. That patients meant more than family as it felt on that Christmas so long ago.

The former patient went on to apologize to my sisters and I while he spoke to the crowd. He said, through tears, that he was sorry he took my father away from his children but that he was so grateful. Wow. At that very moment, all the days my father was late, missed an event, or left too early in the morning for me to say goodbye began to make sense. My lens had changed over the years. Tears welled in my eyes, and I swallowed hard. I loved hearing about my father in this real, raw way. These were people who worked for him, with him, and even a patient of his from a young age who followed in his footsteps and became a burn surgeon. To me, this was the greatest form of flattery. This sort of almost living *eulogy* to my father continued for the next few years. It happened at an award ceremony a few years later. It happened in every letter and email and card and visit from friends and colleagues. It happened when I wrote a piece for the alma mater that my father and I shared, upon his fiftieth reunion.

Once it was time for lunch, I made sure to sit close to the guest of honor. I felt bad he was left to socialize alone. I wanted to be my dad's "wing woman," to navigate conversations with him or for him in case he was tired or overwhelmed by this momentous event, as I seemed to be.

I don't know why I felt he needed my protection or company, but something just seemed vulnerable about him that day. At times, he looked lost since my mother was off talking with friends, so I stepped in to help. He was seated at the head of a long banquet table with a large mirror behind him. He looked out at the sea of faces, and he reminded me of a king surveying his court. Two older, retired colleagues were seated next to each other, and I commented that it was nice to see them, as they had both been recovering from separate bouts of cancer. My father looked up from his meal and, in almost a whisper, said, "Yes. They are doing better, but I'm afraid I might be in for a similar fate." All the noise around me muted. I could hear nothing but the blood pounding in my head. *What did he just say?!?* I looked down at my food. I was no longer hungry. I didn't clarify anything; I physically could not bring myself to respond to my father's comment that caught me off guard and spoiled the rest of the event for me. I was shocked. I was in disbelief. I even questioned what I had just heard. I didn't really want to know. For my father to reference his own health or a *concern* about his own health was absolutely unfamiliar to me. It scared me.

That was the moment I started to watch my father like a hawk. I eyed his every move and physical change and waited for the truth to surface. I honestly wasn't even sure my dad ever saw a physician or had routine physicals. His health history was a mystery, and as far as I knew, he had endured two back surgeries and carried some excess weight but was otherwise healthy. Why would my father say this to me that day and at that moment? Was I supposed to respond? Was that him trying to tell me something was wrong? Instead of pushing him harder for an explanation, I tried to forget what he said. I had waited too long to finally have time with my father that felt normal, free, and without the demands of work; I was not ready to accept anything less. I would not let his comment open the door for anything else. I was selfish and did not want to know anything more. I was like a little girl putting her fingers in her ears, singing loudly to drown out the noise around her.

2

---◆◆◆---

Four months after my dad retired and my parents moved to New Hampshire, Dad and I went skiing for what would be the last time. My dad drove us down the bumpy, hilly road that led from his home to Mount Sunapee at a snail's pace of twenty miles an hour. Looking back on that time, I realize that due to his disease already affecting his comprehension of numbers, he probably couldn't read his speedometer to know what speed he was actually traveling, so he drove by feel. I mentioned a few times that the speed limit was thirty, usually when someone got too close behind, but he just kept his eyes focused on the road. The fifteen-minute ride was mostly quiet, as I admired snow-covered hills in the distance and occasionally glanced at the speedometer to see if he had sped up as I had advised. This had become our winter Wednesday ritual. I would drive to my parents' house early in the morning after getting my oldest, Jacob, off to first grade, and I would bring my two-and-a-half-year-old daughter, Hannah, with me. My mom, never an avid skier, would spend time with her granddaughter while Dad and I skied for a few hours. My dad was sixty-six and still skied. It was remarkable and inspiring. I remember the first time we skied on a Wednesday. I looked at the pricing on the menu and said, "Dad, once you are seventy, the price goes way down for you."

He let out a snort and commented, "Yeah, right. I won't be skiing then."

I responded, "Why not? Of course you will!"

He said a few hours was enough for his old bones, but I still remember a time as a child when we skied from 8 A.M. to 4 P.M. and only rested for twenty minutes for a quick lunch, usually consisting of a yogurt or sandwich, and a quick restroom break. My dad was hardcore, in his work and in his hobbies. Rest was for the weary. Work hard, play hard. My dad had skied almost every major ski mountain in the United States. He had skied every state in the West and took our family along on many ski trips that always were conveniently linked with a surgical meeting over winter or spring break. It was where I saw my dad in a different light. He relaxed around the snow, the mountain air, and the occasional goggle tan. Unlike many skiers, my father never adopted the habit of drinking alcohol while he skied. As I grew into an adult, I never skied and drank either. I followed his lead. I asked him why he never enjoyed a beer on the mountain. His response, as with many of his "teachings," was related to a patient's story. He told me he thought skiing and drinking was "stupid." In his time in Vermont as a young surgeon, he once had to harvest the kidneys of a guy who had been drunk while skiing, hit a tree, and died. That story stuck with me, and I decided I'd rather enjoy skiing sober and keeping my kidneys.

The wind cut through the trees, stinging our faces, and I offered my dad a piece of gum, another ski ritual of ours since I was kid. My dad didn't chew gum often but always did when he skied. On our last day skiing, we mostly skied the green trails—the easiest, flattest trails. I was fine with that, as I wasn't young anymore either, and it was honestly so easy and enjoyable. My dad skied ahead of me, as he always had. He would stop and look up the mountain and wait for me to arrive at his side. My heart was bursting that day. I was skiing with my dad. Life was good. He made the smallest, sharpest, slightest turns on the side of the hill. He was methodical, wise, precise, and always thinking ahead. I imagine this is how he used to operate on his patients as well. I asked him, "Why do you ski like that? All the way over on the side?"

He replied, "The snow is always the best, untouched, people aren't in my way, and I'm not in theirs."

As in his career, he never bragged. He never asked for praise or discussed his skiing unless asked. My father led by example, not words, something I came to see later in life through his illness. He skied half way and waited for me. That day, I skied slower. I slowed down, so his rest was longer. I knew he was most likely pushing himself harder than a man of his age should, and I didn't ever want to embarrass him, so I made sure he had extra time to recoup between runs without making it obvious.

The chairlift was our time to chat. The cold air slowed our speech as we tried to talk with frozen lips, but the fresh air made it worth it. He'd ask about my life; I'd try and ask about his. I remember thinking, *Now is the time to ask him whatever you've always wanted to know about his career, his childhood, his thoughts.* Our skiing time was our bonding time. It was just the two of us. This was what I had been waiting so many years for, this chance to just *be* with my dad, to get to know him as a person, as a man. I hung on my dad's every word. I felt that all his wisdom was like gold, to be cherished and kept close. He had an answer for everything. I was looking forward to many more ski days and conversations over the coming years, so I could finally feel close with my father. I wish, back then, that he had let me in on what was happening to him. I wish I had known that my time with him like this was short. By the following February, I would give birth to another child, and my dad and I would never again make plans to ski together.

3

It was one year later, and I was nearing the end of my pregnancy. My son Henry's birth was scheduled for February 25th by C-section. The plans were made. My parents would take the kids the night before, and Denis and I would head to the hospital, well-rested and showered, early on the morning of the 25th to welcome our third and final child.

Instead, Henry decided he was in charge. Shortly after midnight on February 17th, while an ice storm raged outside my window, I was awoken by a feeling of warm liquid between my legs. My eyes popped open after registering what had just happened, and I immediately sat up and rolled out of bed. "Denis, I think my water just broke!" I waddled to the bathroom and felt my first contraction and, with it, more liquid. Denis followed me to the bathroom, squinting from the light I had flipped on in a flurry of panic while shouting for the phone to call the hospital. Each birth was different for my children, and this circumstance warranted some direction from my doctor. Though this wasn't my first time having my water break, it didn't take long for me to confirm that I was, indeed, in labor, and my doctor instructed me to get to the hospital as soon as possible. I phoned my parents around 1:30 A.M. to report the change in plans and deliver the surprising news of the impending birth, ahead of schedule. I managed to have the conversation while I worked my way around the room, throwing clothes in a bag. I had never packed my "go" bag, thinking I had plenty of time left, as Henry was still two weeks from his actual due date. Denis showered, and I contracted every few minutes. When I called my parents, my father answered the phone. This was something that was old hat for him—a phone call in the middle of the night relaying unexpected medical news. When he answered, he seemed shocked, even confused. I expected him to go straight into doctor mode, as he often did. Months prior, I experienced a scare regarding an exposure to a potentially dangerous virus for my unborn baby. I panicked and called my dad to ask him his opinion, more so to put my mind at ease. "I'm sure you already had that illness as a child. Almost all people have had it by adulthood," he told me with an assurance of a doctor and the sensitivity of the dad I had needed that day. I took a huge breath and sighed. I was so grateful to have a dad who was a doctor. It was free, trusted, medical advice. And, as always, he was right. I was immune, as the blood test showed days later.

That night, instead of asking me how I was or triaging my labor as I might have hoped, he immediately said, with a tiredness and quiver to his voice, "Here. Talk to Mom." My moment of excitement about sharing my news and meeting my baby, his grandchild, faded at his seemingly dismissive response.

I explained to my mother that I needed to head to the hospital right away because the baby was coming now, and I still needed a C-section. Unfortunately, living forty-five minutes away from each other in an ice storm didn't bode well for my parents to race right over. She said they would be down in a few hours. I was a little disappointed but tried to understand. Sometimes things don't work out like you plan. We called Denis's sister who lived twenty minutes away, and she made it over within forty minutes, dodging icy branches and navigating slippery roads. She arrived like a fairy godmother, and I was so grateful, as my contractions had started to pick up. Talking through them was getting to be more difficult, which history and many Google searches over my eight-year stint with pregnancy and motherhood, has told me was time to go.

Henry was born two hours later by C-section, without incident, while his brother and sister slept, blissfully unaware of the chaos that had ensued down the hall. By 6 A.M., my parents had arrived to relieve the fairy godmother of her duties, and the children finally came downstairs to hear the news that they had gained a brother overnight. Later that morning, my parents brought the kids to meet Henry, and when they arrived, my father looked horrible. His eyes looked washed over with exhaustion and a touch of sadness, or maybe worry. Which then made me worry. I didn't want to have to worry about him or anyone else that day. I wanted to just enjoy my new baby. He congratulated me and came over to catch a glance of Henry, but when it came time to hold him, only my mother did while my father looked on. The same man who, when Jacob, his first grandson, was born, bowled me over to get into the house, while exclaiming, "Where is he? I want to see my grandson!" He was the proudest, happiest grandfather, always telling his nurses and patients about his grandkids and sharing pictures. But on the day of Henry's birth, I could see something in his eyes that was almost vacant. He was wearing an old pair of glasses because, according to my mother, he lost or broke his other pair. I could not pinpoint what was different, but I knew something was gone—a light had started to fade. I had only seen this look once, and it had been a few months before. He had driven down to my house with my mother, only to arrive with a blurred look in his eyes. Solemn. Tired. After visiting only a few short hours, he expressed interest, as well as concern, with needing to go home. He commented, "Let's get home before dark." It was at least three hours before sunset, but he was ready to go. It annoyed me— almost hurt me—that he didn't want to spend more time together. In later years, I realized that this was probably part of his disease, causing him to be anxious and most likely not able to grasp the concept of time anymore. I forgave him for this. I tried to stop taking it personally, as it continued with the progression of his disease, and it would occur during visits to other places, not just my home.

I sat in my hospital bed with conflicting emotions. I was so full of love that Henry had arrived that morning safely and met his brother and sister. My children were excited, Denis was a proud father of three, and my parents were both here to witness the event. My family felt complete, whole. Yet, while I sat there holding Henry to my chest and smiling, I felt that nagging anxiety deep inside. What was wrong with Dad? I had pure joy, love, and a deep concern, all at the same time. As a mother, I knew this feeling well. However, as a daughter, this was new for me. I had gained a boy in my life that day but felt I was slowly losing a man.

4

Henry's birth was a great distraction for my family. Having a new baby brought an excitement and nervous energy to our house and family. Most of my thoughts were consumed by the baby's eating, diaper changing, sleeping, and crying. When Henry was a few weeks old, he developed a hemangioma, a type of rosy, raised birthmark in his gluteal cleft. I thought it was just diaper rash. After his primary care physician saw him, she quickly referred me to dermatology for further examination. I didn't think much of it—a skin issue—*okay, we can handle that*. The appointment with dermatology took a drastic turn, as I was warned that the location of his hemangioma could indicate a much bigger problem. This type and location meant Henry could have urinary, bowel, or even walking issues. It meant he could have a tethered spinal cord and may require surgery. My world imploded. My sweet, perfect, little newborn could have devastating complications for the rest of his life. I was in shock. Denis had not come with me that day, and I was terrified to hear this news and process it alone. I, of course, called my father. He was calm and reassuring, yet on guard. He assured me Henry was being seen at a wonderful hospital, but if Henry required surgery or a second opinion, we would go to Boston, the Mecca of all children's health needs. I felt protected and safe. I had my dad in my corner.

Dad asked to accompany me to Henry's dermatology appointment when his hemangioma had subsequently ulcerated. It became an open sore and needed wound treatment, something my father had been a leading expert in for years. He was quiet in the appointment, playing more the part of grandfather and father, but I have no doubt he was playing doctor in his head and watching over what was being recommended. I felt so safe that day with him there. As we left the appointment, he chimed in to the resident who saw us that day, "I used to do this for a living."

"Oh, were you a doctor?" the resident replied.

"Yeah, I was, for about forty years," my father said with a small smile and the tiniest chuckle. He didn't share that working with skin was his life's work. Why didn't he share more? The connection of who he was never was made, as my father and I did not share a last name. His name was only "Dad" or "Papa" in the exam room that day. When I looked back in Henry's medical record and read the notes, it stated, "Henry presents today with mother and grandfather." I think seeing that label in writing would have made my father proud had he seen it then. It made me proud to read it and have him be known as just my child's grandfather, a role I was so happy he was taking in our lives post-retirement. Henry's medical issue seemed to bring a little life back to my father. Maybe he felt needed or felt like he needed to be there for me, but it seemed to work. My dad had brightened a bit and seemed more focused for those few months of uncertainty surrounding Henry's health. When Henry was finally cleared of any serious medical condition, by May of that year, we all breathed a sigh of relief. My father must have decided that after that was resolved, we could handle more news.

5

O ctober in New England is my favorite time of year. The leaves in New Hampshire are a colorful pattern of green, orange, yellow, and red, the air is crisp, and we begin to fall into a patchwork world full of pumpkins, witches, ghosts, turkeys, and sweaters. Henry was a thriving, bald cherub who was finally weaned and sleeping somewhat through the night. Jacob and Hannah were used to having a baby in the house and were busy with learning to read or losing teeth, and Denis and I were settling into being outnumbered, yet content and complete.

Amy flew in for a visit, and Liza made the drive from Boston to stay at my parents. My mother called me and requested a dinner out with the family. "Maybe just me, Dad, your sisters, and you would be nice," she said to me a few days before Amy's arrival. She didn't have to ask me twice; I was happy to spend a dinner out not worrying about my children, able to feel like an adult only and not a mother too. In typical fashion, my sisters and I discussed attire and cooed and hugged when we finally were together at my parents' house, shortly before dinner. We made the ten-minute drive to the small, cozy downtown area. It was a classic New England town, complete with sidewalks, cafes, artisan shops, and a small college with a white church with a steeple.

We ordered a bottle of wine, and after we all had a few sips and had placed our orders, my mother looked at us all and said, "Dad and I brought you here tonight because it's time one of us sees a doctor."

"What?!? What's going on?" There were gasps from my sisters and I and probably an "Oh God" uttered from at least two of us. I immediately thought, *Oh no. Mom has cancer or lymphoma.* My mother has an autoimmune disease that can lead to this as it progresses. My face got hot with worry, and my heart started to pound. I looked to my dad, who didn't say a word.

My mother continued, "It's not me, girls. There is something wrong with your father. He's asked to see a doctor." The room muted. I stared at my dad to see if I could identify exactly what was wrong with him. I searched his face for something—anything. My dad had been losing weight, a lot of it. My mother always said he was "trying to," but I didn't believe her. My paternal grandfather had died at the young age of seventy-three from complications of leukemia, and I wondered if this would also be my father's fate, ever since that day at the retirement party. Little did I know it wasn't my grandfather's fate but rather my late grandmother's fate that was in store for my dad.

Amy pushed with the questions, "What is it? Why? What's going on?"

"He can't tell time anymore," my mother said with a gentleness and whisper to her voice.

"Dad, is this true?" Amy directed her mouth straight at him.

I was speechless again as I had been that day at the retirement party. This conversation was unfolding before my eyes, and I was frozen. If I didn't say anything, maybe it wouldn't happen or become real. I also felt if I addressed my father directly, I would embarrass him or force him to admit something he wasn't ready to do. I let everyone speak around me. The voices swirled around me like a swarm of black flies on a mid-May day in New Hampshire. My father nodded his head slowly and immediately looked to my mother to speak on his behalf, something that had

33

become a more obvious behavior in the last few months. I felt my view of my father, the all-knowing, powerful, verbose, and successful surgeon, begin to narrow. I focused on him, and everything else blurred around me. He was like a little lost child at the end of a tunnel with a spotlight shining on him. He seemed smaller all of a sudden—weak, frail, and vulnerable. His body had considerably shrunk over the last few years, and he was at the lowest weight I had ever known him to be. I felt a vulnerability from him that I had never witnessed in my thirty-seven years on Earth. Aside from the two back surgeries, my father was never sick; he never even had a sniffle. The back surgeries came twenty-five years into his career and at the expense of it. He operated to save lives while continuing to inflict damage on his own body for the love of his craft.

Amy's PhD in neuroscience kicked into high gear. Amy started listing neurological disorders, and I remember her saying the word "aphasia."

"What is that?" I finally spoke as if I had snapped out of a trance.

"It's a speech issue," she replied without looking at me.

My mind began to race, and I began to think—*it's a*

brain tumor, cancer, or a stroke. I had no MD or PhD after my name, but a million thoughts began to enter my mind. Like a round table of doctors, we all sat discussing what it could be while my father maintained his silence, nodding his head every so often. A man who normally led groups of medical students, residents, and colleagues sat back and listened, and as a good doctor does, he did not offer a diagnosis or an idea until he had more information.

"We are going to see our primary care doctor next week; we will see what he says. We will start there," my mother said firmly, while reaching for my father's hand.

The fact he was submitting to a visit with a doctor was serious. One of my first fears was coming true. The fear that my parents, specifically my father, needed medical help or worse, die. The man whom we always looked to for medical advice, support, or a vote of confidence was now staring back at us in his vulnerability and subtle fear. If Dad needed help, what did that mean for us? He was always our strong foundation.

Our dinner continued, and the wine flowed, along with tears of worry and concern. I don't remember anything I ate that night; my appetite had disappeared. Eating a good meal after receiving that news felt wrong and almost disrespectful. I felt selfish and upset that my dad's health was why we were brought there that night, but I immediately wiped that feeling away and replaced it with sadness. Our family was changing before my eyes. My mother stepped into a role of managing my father's healthcare that night, and it was daunting. My father always managed my mother's healthcare, not the reverse. This was uncharted territory —for my mother and for our family to witness this role reversal. My mother appeared to be up for the challenge, at least that night at dinner. She sat taller, more confident, and ready for a battle. She was a warrior, and my father needed *her* protection this time. Witnessing that made my world feel off kilter. The doctor became the patient, and it scared the crap out of me. I felt as if I was in a house of mirrors where everything looked distorted and people run around frightened, trying to find a normal mirror to see what they are used to seeing.

6

My mother called around six o'clock on the evening of my father's appointment with his primary care physician. Her first words came out with a quiet sigh, "Oh, Andrea. It's bad. It's really bad news." My mother had always held down the fort. She was the one we confided in, cried to, yelled at, complained to, depended on, and felt closest to. She spent her days chasing after us, cleaning, cooking, shuttling us to and from school and activities, all while attempting to maintain volunteer positions and be a surgeon's wife. In 1990, when I was eleven, she was the one to tell my sisters and me that we were moving to Chicago, so my dad could accept a position as a director of the burn and shock trauma unit at a major hospital. She was the one who told me when my paternal grandfather died in 1993, and now she was the one to tell me more devastating news.

I immediately broke out in a cold sweat, and my heart began to pound. Tunnel vision took over.

"What? What is it?" I spat out as fast as I could.

"The doctor says your father has dementia. He gave him a test, and your father failed it. He is cognitively impaired, somewhat significantly," my mother said in a calm, quiet voice.

Oh. My. God. No! This is not possible. How? My father was a genius, he was an eloquent speaker, he knew something about everything, and dementia was for *old* people. No, this couldn't be right. It must be a brain tumor. I felt sick to my stomach. I felt vulnerable and alone. I denied what my mother was telling me, saying to myself, *The doctor doesn't know what he is talking about; he doesn't know my dad.*

"So, what's next? What do we do now?!?" My voice came out with an urgency, and my throat was dry.

"Well, he recommended we see a neurologist," my mother said gently, but I could hear her sadness and disappointment. Her world just crashed down around her that day.

I paused and then it hit me. "What did Dad say? What does he think?" I hadn't even thought of *his* reaction to all of this.

"He was very quiet. He really didn't say anything, but he knows he wants to spend time with his family as much as he can. He also doesn't want anyone to know about this right now. He has his pride," my mother responded.

"Is it Alzheimer's like Memere had?" My paternal grandmother, lovingly termed Memere, which was French for grandmother, had only died two years prior due to Alzheimer's at age eighty-nine. How could her son, at only sixty-seven, be diagnosed already?

"We don't know that yet. He will need further testing to determine the cause, to see whether it is truly dementia and not a brain tumor or something else causing his cognitive impairment," my mother said flatly. I wondered if she said these words with as much numbing shock as I heard them.

Okay, so there was hope it could be a brain tumor that could shrink, be removed, or treated. It could be something that would get better and go away. Somehow, this diagnosis seemed more acceptable, more palatable, and, in a way, less embarrassing for my family and for my dad. There was no way my father had Alzheimer's. That meant he would forget things, and he never forgot things. For years, my mother said my father had a photographic memory, and, other than possibly not knowing my actual birth date (a long-running family joke), he knew everything. Soon, his own birth date ended up eluding him, and his own age often came as a surprise to him when we reminded him, among other things.

"When is the appointment with the neurologist?" I asked. I hoped it was already scheduled, maybe for tomorrow. *Wasn't this an emergency?*

"Next month. Sometime in December," my mother replied.

We ended the call with a thick melancholy hanging over us. We both said "I love you," a phrase that we never used lightly in my family. A phrase that really meant, "I'm with you on this; you aren't alone." When we said it, we meant it. The sun had already set a few hours before, and I could see my reflection in a nearby window. Everything felt different. The lights in the house seemed wrong. I needed to turn on more to brighten the darkness I could feel trying to extinguish the light, the darkness that was trying to convince me the sun wouldn't rise again.

I cried the rest of the night. I googled for three hours, listened to sad music, and read what might be next for my father. My heart was broken. It felt as if my dad had died; the man I knew was gone. My father crashed down that day from the pedestal I had placed him on. I couldn't figure out what I was feeling and then I realized he seemed more human to me that day, the day of his initial diagnosis, than he ever had been. My father was stoic, untouchable at times—often emotionally, but more so physically, as he was always working or traveling and elusive. I spent most of my childhood with my father trying to get closer to him, to feel accepted by him, and to know him. Maybe it was his training as a surgeon or his constant time away from home, but my father was a private, closed man for the most part and only in special instances, or ones of pure surprise, did I gain insight into who he was or what he was thinking behind those glasses. He was the patriarchal father figure, who was raised by a first-generation Italian World War II veteran from Massachusetts and a French-Canadian dairy farmer from Vermont. He ruled his three daughters with a strict, firm upbringing but always with a softness, especially if we came to him confused and in tears about failing chemistry or having to build a science project. My father could build, repair, clean, and maintain anything. He had the mind of MacGyver and the motivation of the Energizer Bunny. It was inspiring, as much as it was exhausting, to be his daughter.

My first time skiing, he didn't put me in a lesson or on the bunny hill. He put skis on me, handed me my polls, and up we went on the chairlift. I was a terrified six-year-old being led by an overly confident father, but he continued the same message throughout my life. Be cautious, trust yourself, don't screw up, and have confidence that you can do this, even if you don't think you can yet. My first time driving, he took me on a side road near our home and told me not to look behind me and just drive—to trust myself. He had more confidence in me than I ever had in myself. His own confidence was quiet, humble, and never discussed. The only time I remember him referencing his own success was in a passing story he shared with my mother one day after work. Apparently, a patient's family had questioned him on his knowledge and expertise to care for their loved one. According to the story and what I remember, he just looked at them and said, "Just look me up on the internet," and walked away—my guess is, along with a smirk and maybe even a chuckle. My guess also is that they never brought it up again, as they more than likely learned he was one of the best, if not *the* best, surgeons in the country, possibly the world, to care for their loved one. It was evident in the positions he held, the societies he was a member and often president of, and his position as editor in chief of a burn journal. He was the director of a research lab, the chairman of surgery, the dean of the medical school, eventually the provost and senior vice president, and he earned numerous awards and honors, locally, domestically, and internationally. He didn't need to remind anyone in the medical world who he was. He was a master, a giant, a god to some. He was a man to be admired, sometimes feared, but most of all, respected. That night, he became human, vulnerable, sick, dependent, and, most of all, mortal.

I struggled to make sense of the news I had gotten that week. I continued to search Google endlessly and read about all the stages and phases my father could and eventually would enter. The idea of it was terrifying. How would I be able to handle seeing this happen? When would it happen? Tomorrow? Next month? In three years? Maybe he would just linger in this mild cognitive impairment for a while, and life would continue as normal, yet with one eye always watching him. Donald Trump was elected President, and my father was diagnosed with dementia. The world felt very backward. I commented often that it felt like *The Twilight Zone*. I had been stung twice that summer by bees and ended up in the emergency room due to a potential allergy. This year was ending on a low note. Henry's birth was the only upside to that year for me, and even with that came some unexpected challenges. One night, Denis came home from work, and I couldn't keep it together. The kids were watching TV, and I just burst into tears. Denis took me in his arms, and I sobbed. I finally said, "It's not fair! My father spent his whole life helping people, saving lives, and now this, and no one and nothing will save him!" Denis just hugged me and let me cry. Then, he started to cry too and simply replied, "I know." *Thank God for Denis.*

My coping mechanism was usually to find the positive in a negative situation—to search out the reason from the well-known statement "everything happens for a reason." When I had miscarried a few years before, twice in six months, I rationalized it with not being the right timing; I trusted in God's plan. I learned from my misfortune and hopefully helped friends with the same experience. This time, I could not find my reason. I could not see the light at the end of the tunnel. I could not rationalize my father's diagnosis. I didn't know what to say to him the next time I saw him. There was no positive. My expectations of the future were bleak. My dreams for my father and me to have a better, closer relationship were dashed. My father, the way I knew him, had begun to fade away from me; my view had started to change. If his memory was going to slowly disappear, what would be left for me, for my family? What *would* remain? My beautiful painting of the future had been ruined as if someone had dumped water all over it, and the colors ran together in a muddled mess, and nothing was clear anymore.

7

My father had his MRI a few days later, and no brain tumor was found. It further clarified his diagnosis was actually dementia and that he experienced a small TIA, a stroke, at one point. Regardless, whatever was destroying his brain could not be cured or removed. It was there to stay. My sisters and I discussed, at length on the phone or over text, our opinions and feelings on the subject. We were close and texted daily, often mundane things, but our connection was solid, and we were sisters who had become friends. Amy's neuroscience background and subsequent work in the pharmaceutical industry offered us a scientific approach, and Liza's social work background in the field of burns, just like my dad, was often helpful as well.

While we were close as adults, we had grown up with times of separation. Amy started college while Liza entered fifth grade, and so much of their relationship had been big sister and little sister stuff, like babysitting or driving her around. Amy and I were nearer in age but fought like cats. Once Amy went off to college, we became closer. Maybe it was maturity or the absence of each other that eventually drew us together. Amy, being highly intelligent and more apt to be found buried in a book, answered me in a few words. She reminded me of Dad. She thought over what she was going to say before she said it, and it was typically profound and usually right. Liza was more like me and emotionally driven, but still diplomatic in her responses. Her profession in social work was perfect for her, as she was often the peacemaker or the go-between in the family. The three of us were often at very different places in our lives while living under the same roof due to our eight-year age span. We fought over the TV, the bathroom, and who got the front seat in the car. We didn't hang out together, as we had different interests and friends. When we were young, our age gap seemed like an entire lifetime, but as we aged, the gap tightened and eventually, we were all in our twenties, post-college, and diving into life, and things felt more balanced between us. We hadn't all lived in the same state since I was fifteen, but that didn't stop us from remaining close. We were in each other's weddings, Amy is my oldest son, Jacob's, godmother, Liza babysat my children for weekends away, and we all shared a strong love for each other, our parents, and their well-being. Whether it was a phone call, an email, a text, or a Facebook picture, we were in constant communication. Our parents fostered our relationship as sisters and as a family of five, gathering us for holidays, family vacations, or other special events throughout the years.

My sisters embraced Denis like a brother when he and I met when I was nineteen and in college in Vermont. They often defended him to me when I complained about something I didn't like or a fight we had. My sisters loving Denis always comforted me. It also validated I had married the right one. My sister's opinions were ones I often sought out first and were, many times, the most important. I knew they would be honest, and, most of all, I trusted them. They were the most like me in the whole world, with shared parents and a past, and they knew me well. We had similar features that linked us as sisters—our eyes, our smiles, and our brown hair, but all still having our own unique look. Amy had straight hair, Liza had an abundance of curls, and I fell somewhere in the middle, both with height and hair, with my waves that came out in the humidity. I didn't shy away from sharing all aspects of my life with my sisters, so often times, they didn't have a choice to know things about me. They weren't as apt to share all the details from their lives on a regular basis, but if something felt worthy, they would. I knew when Amy was having trouble in her first marriage, I knew when Liza was dating a guy in college, and they knew every detail of my pregnancies and most of my inner thoughts and worries about everything and anything.

We still argued and disagreed at times, but we quickly moved past things, as we knew how important our relationship was to maintain as adults. Our arguments were never beyond something somewhat trivial, such as someone feeling left out of a conversation or someone being misunderstood for the way they phrased a statement. We had learned to address it openly as adults, sending a text or asking directly, "Are you upset with me about something?" We had seen too many sibling relationships fall apart around us. We were committed to being open and honest with each other. As my dad's illness progressed, we started to learn to depend on one another for emotional support beyond the typical day-to-day, "Does this shirt look okay on me?" type questions. We texted each other often sharing our thoughts, theories, and feelings about Dad's recent diagnosis. Mostly, we shared our sadness. We all felt the same. Lost. Confused. Worried.

My father declined any further testing following his MRI, rigorous testing that lasted hours and closely scrutinized his mental capabilities. He declined a trip to Boston to see other specialists. My father was resigned to his diagnosis and was continuing to decline. He often said, when questioned about seeing other doctors, "I don't want to be a guinea pig. I know what they will do, and I don't want that." He also declined any medication, knowing, as a doctor, the side effects and what they may bring. I tried to reason with my mother. "What if we just tried another doctor? A trip to Boston to see what they think?"

She pushed back, "It's not what your dad wants." I agreed and then changed my mind the next day. I walked a line between respecting my father's wishes and being damn mad that he didn't want to fight this. *Why didn't he want to help himself? How could he just accept this?* He had access to the best healthcare, some would say, in the country. Why didn't he want to go to Boston as he had wanted to for Henry? This was a time that his medical degree was possibly a detriment to himself. He knew what the medicines and tests meant, what they involved. He didn't like that idea. He didn't want to be a test subject or just a number. He still had the upper hand in his own health. The decision was ultimately his to make, and an educated one at that.

Eventually, the neurologist agreed that any medication would not help him at that point, regardless. The only options he had were how he chose to spend his remaining time. As a daughter and a bystander in this process, essentially, I struggled to accept my father's resignation to his diagnosis. I started to see that spending my energy trying to get him to do something I thought he should do was a waste. I needed to put my energy into making the best of the time we had together, time that began to feel shorter and shorter each day.

8

---◆──◆──◆---

Two months after his diagnosis, my dad was set to receive an award in Vermont. He was being honored with an inaugural achievement from the university, appropriately named the Catamount Surgeon Award. It was particularly special for my father to receive an award from the institution where he had been a medical student, a resident, and eventually an attending until our big move to Chicago. Our family was so proud, but after his diagnosis, a shadow was cast. Doubt was cast in my mother's mind about my father being able to attend and accept the award comfortably, in an appropriate manner— appropriate meaning as his old self, one who couldn't be identified as having dementia. His diagnosis was still private, only known by my family. It was still considered top secret at that time. My father had lost eighty pounds over the prior two years and looked healthy, yet his mind was not. He could carry a conversation but often skipped around words, using more general terms, rather than the eloquent or complicated terms he used in years past. He would also turn a question into a question. "Dad, what do you want for dinner?" He would respond by saying, "Well, what do you want?" He did this with menus—he would say, "What's good here?" It was most likely a cover for, "I can't make out this confusing menu." My sisters and I convinced my mother it was okay for Dad to go to Vermont. The trip was about a two-hour ride and an overnight stay in a hotel. I think he also wanted to go and was still very physically independent, so it was now or never.

It was another event where past colleagues discussed my father's career. An old friend and colleague spoke lovingly and wonderfully about my father as an early resident and, later, an attending. I fought back tears hearing these memories. He described moments that happened before I even made my appearance in my father's life. He told us about my dad, the young doctor; it was a time I was never privy to. What happened within those hospital walls made my father the man I came to know. The colleague spoke of things I always imagined as a daughter of a doctor, but to hear other doctors say them of him was awe-inspiring. My father's legacy at the hospital was still alive and well. It was this same colleague who had performed successful surgeries on both of my grandparents, as well as my mother-in-law, so to have him not only save the lives of people I love, but to also speak so admirably of my father, was truly extraordinary. With my father's recently diagnosed illness, those words were even sweeter. Bittersweet. I loved hearing those stories. At some moments, especially then, it felt as if his eulogy was being given to him directly—while he was still alive, while he could still remember, while *we* could still remember. It was a wonderful trip down memory lane for my family. The event took place at the same country club where I had my wedding reception thirteen years before. It was now a place of celebration, new life, old life, happiness, and tears.

Then it came time for my father's acceptance speech. I took a deep breath. My heart began to race, even though I had a glass of wine to calm my nerves. My father had nothing written down. This was typical for him to speak off-the-cuff, to speak from his genius mind and deep heart. He walked up to the podium, a man half the size of what he was when he was that maverick of a resident, once upon a time, who we had just heard about. He thanked the crowd and the university. He used words like "team" and "group." Over and over again. He did his best. He fooled everyone. He did it. He carried off a speech in front of nearly one hundred people, two months after being diagnosed with dementia. He was incredible. I cried because I was proud. I cried because I was saddened that my joy was being clouded by the awful secret we kept. That was the last time my father spoke to a crowd. How fitting. The place where he began his career in medicine was the same place he ended it, being honored with recognition.

It was in the state and town where my family began. The place my parents met and fell in love and had three daughters. The place I met my husband and fell in love and got married. The place my father spent countless hours studying, writing, researching, teaching, and operating. Blood, sweat, and tears, literally. Vermont was our home. It was a place I wanted to always go back to; it was a warm blanket on a cold day for me. It was my heart.

On the morning we left to head back to New Hampshire, I looked out the hotel window at the frozen lake and the Adirondacks across the way. Gorgeous, yet ominous. Winter had arrived and wouldn't relent for months. Our family was about to endure a winter as well. Snowstorms crept in. The weatherman said it was coming. One snowflake at a time, the skies grew darker, and the clouds hung like puffy gray cotton. But, like a winter storm, it's never known exactly how it will play out. Will the wind get crazy and knock down a tree and turn out the lights? Will the snow fall quietly, gently coating the ground, and be still? Will it be heavy and wet and hard to move? Will it be light and fluffy and blow away with slight wind? Will it melt the next day and reveal green grass below it, still struggling to survive? My dad's diagnosis was like that winter storm forecast. It was going to happen, but storms are unpredictable, and you can only prepare so much. You have to sit back and wait for the snow to fall and huddle close to those you love, hoping the storm doesn't destroy all in its wake.

9

The first time my mom called to report a significant change in my father made my heart sink. We knew he couldn't tell time looking at a watch or a clock with hands, but my mother then commented that he was having trouble writing. He was forgetting how. *This is really happening,* I thought. My father was eight months into his diagnosis and had already been attending speech therapy for a few months. It was brutal for him, as he struggled to write even a sentence for his homework, which was to journal or answer a question. My mother expressed that it sometimes took hours for him to get down a thought on paper. It was almost as if his brain couldn't tell his hands what to do. Not only did he struggle to form a thought, but the actual art of writing was beginning to be lost on him. The forming of letters and motor skills was disappearing. My dad had mild cognitive impairment at that point, but it seemed to be getting worse. Only about a year before, my father could still use his computer and type an email. Though handwriting was never his strong suit, my mother had noticed a sharp decline in his ability to use pen and paper, compared to months before when he had attempted to keep a journal.

His speech was somewhat limited, but he could still carry a conversation and was aware of his surroundings. He was able to eat and walk, but dressing himself became increasingly harder. He often woke early in the morning, around four o'clock, to dress himself, and he sometimes told my mother he had patients to see or a meeting to attend. He had been retired for almost three years at that point. My mother said she would find clothes strewn about in my dad's closet after these early wake-ups. He would be wearing a shirt or pair of pants backward, and my mother gently, patiently, would guide him back to bed or to the living room to rest while she got herself ready for the day. He didn't argue or fight her on her attempts to distract and dissuade him from his missions, or what he believed to be his missions. That early morning confusion happened often and was definitely a time that he was not lucid or aware of his current state of reality and illness. My mother's voice and words were enough to draw him back into some sort of "here and now" moment. He would listen and it would eventually snap him out of his almost trancelike state, and he would sit down and wait for her to turn on the TV or get him breakfast.

I never witnessed this early morning confusion, but my mother called me almost daily to report the newest phase or symptom my father seemed to be experiencing. It wasn't unusual for us to talk daily before my father's diagnosis, but it was becoming the focus. Depending on my own stress levels for the day or my schedule, these calls could serve to either distract me from my own challenges with my children or add to my increasing anxiety about my father's well-being. "Well, your father turned on all the lights early this morning while trying to find clothes to wear. I'm exhausted and it's only 8 A.M.," my mother said during one of our calls, exasperation and a twinge of sadness in her voice. Old Dad, the dad he was before dementia, was so conscious of his actions that when he woke early to get dressed as a working man, he used a flashlight to find his socks in a drawer so as not to disturb my mother's sleep.

My dad surprised us in other ways too. He said hello to complete strangers in public. It was kind, but not the dad I knew who usually kept to himself unless spoken to first. When Dad and I went to the store once to get a few things, I unloaded the cart onto the belt, and the checkout girl looked at me and then my dad. My dad must have thought she needed an explanation for our relation to one another, so he gladly offered one. That is not anything he ever would have done as Old Dad. My dad said, "That's my daughter!" with a smile. I laughed but also felt a bit sad. It wasn't the same dad I used to know. I always sort of wished my dad was warmer and more outspoken to strangers when I was younger, but when it started to happen, it just felt out of character for him. His personality was changing, maybe for the better, but it was foreign to me. It was as if I was getting to know an entirely new person. I enjoyed my father becoming more social in public, but it also made my heart hurt a little. I knew it wasn't his personality; it was his disease that had changed him. I looked at it in a positive light for the most part, as he wasn't rude or inappropriate. He just wasn't the typical stoic, private man I had been used to for so many years. Or maybe he was just letting out a part of himself that had lain dormant for so many years due to his career. He had an innocence about him now that was refreshing, yet also made me want to protect him more than ever. I didn't want him to become someone people saw as vulnerable and able to be taken advantage of due to his kindness. I had heard about older people being convinced to hand over their money or sign up for things they didn't fully understand, and I didn't want my dad to become one of them. I was hypersensitive to his disease affecting his capabilities to make appropriate decisions, and I could feel myself changing from daughter to guardian at those times. We were lucky my father was mellowing. He began appreciating the simple things in life, and he was, from what I could see, content. I had heard stories of people with dementia getting angry or violent, but not my dad.

My father's anxiety also increased, mostly concerning my mother. If they were apart, he worried. Sometimes when I would take him out to pick up lunch or run an errand he would say, "We should get back. Mom is going to worry," or simply, "Mom is worried." Looking back, I also wonder if he couldn't grasp the concept of how much time had passed since we last saw her. My sisters also noticed this when they spent time with my dad. He was always worried about Mom, but I think he felt safest with her. I think his worry wasn't if *she* was okay, but rather, *he* wasn't okay without her. It was sweet and annoying, all at the same time. I constantly reminded him and convinced him that Mom was fine or okay and that she didn't need him to be back right away. It started to affect our time spent together. I felt limited on how long he actually enjoyed my company before he started to get hyper focused on seeing my mother again. I started to anticipate this anxiety and occasionally just offered up details about when we would see Mom again, or that I knew he wanted to get back. I started to employ methods I had used a lot with my kids by reassuring him and trying to observe his body language if he seemed anxious. His needs had become more basic, and his ability to function had become more compromised.

The first time I saw my father wear his clothing wrong was humbling. I went to visit one day, and when I walked in to say hello, my eyes immediately shot to his shirt. The collar of the long sleeve, green T-shirt sat right below the base of his throat, and I could make out the faint outline of the tag. My father's retirement had brought a change of "uniform." Suits and ties were replaced with jeans and long sleeve shirts or sweatshirts. I had a rush of cold sweat run through me out of embarrassment for my dad. This was *real.* I stood a few feet across from him while I hung my purse on the back of the dining room chair. I removed my coat, looked down, and attempted to busy myself while processing what I had just seen. *Oh, Dad.*

Damn, I thought sullenly, as I straightened my own shirt and hiked up my jeans higher on my hips. What else could I do to pass these moments of pure panic and sadness for my father? There were times I pretended life was back to Old Dad, and nothing was different, but this was an obvious time that I could not simply push away what was happening to him. No one chose on purpose to wear their clothing backward, especially my father. He was a man who, in the past, prided himself on his abundance of clothing, cleanliness, and attention to every detail down to cufflinks. My mother must have missed it that morning, or he put it on right before I got there, so she didn't have time to notice. I knew I had two choices. I could either completely ignore it, or I could find a way to point it out to him without making a huge deal of it. His backward shirt glared at me like hazard lights on a car pulled over on the side of the road. I couldn't just drive on past.

I chose to meet that new challenge, rather than pretend I didn't see it. I dove right in and said to myself, *It's now or never*. I knew someone else, like my parents' cleaning lady or one of my children, could see it or point it out, and I wanted to be the one to do it. I wanted to be the one to deliver this news to him without laughing or making him feel bad. If my children noticed it first, they may not have been as gentle with the delivery of the news, probably saying something like, "Papa, you look silly! Why is your shirt on wrong?" I knew how blunt and truthful kids can be. I couldn't bear the thought of my kids hurting my dad's feelings; at the same time, I really had no idea how my father would process that news, but I didn't feel like finding out.

"Dad, here. Come here." I reached out and sort of tapped his collar. "Here, let's just turn this around. I like this shirt. It looks great on you." I tried to pair a negative with a positive, something I had learned as a manager in my "past life" of working. Before Jacob was born, I worked at a student loan company, and at a young age was promoted to manager. I had a few conferences where we learned effective managerial strategies, and that is one I remember clearly. They had explained that delivering bad news or criticism was meant to be like a sandwich. The bread was the good news, and in between was the more difficult news or criticism. I just delivered a sandwich to my father and hoped it didn't leave a bad taste in his mouth.

He looked down. Then, he looked up and sort of smiled at me. He didn't really respond, but he helped pull his shirt over and turn it around. Done. No more talk was needed about that. We could move on. I cried on my way home that day, but not in front of my dad. I'm not sure if it was denial or acceptance that kept me from talking about it more with him. His deficits were probably pointed out enough to him as he struggled to do the things he used to do. I didn't need to add to it.

I realized I needed to take on a new role with my father. I now had to look out for him. My mothering instinct had replaced my instinct as a daughter. I mastered taking care of toddlers and babies, and now I had to learn to care for someone older. It was the first of many times I had to address a difficult and seemingly embarrassing situation for my dad. Another time, as we got ready to leave the house, he put his boots on the wrong feet. I froze when I realized it. All I could think was that was what my kids did when they were two or three. They were able to put them on but didn't have the skill to pick the correct foot. My father was now in that same mindset. Another defeat. Another skill lost. I wilted inside, but I didn't let him see my disappointment or sadness. I just addressed it in a matter-of-fact way. It was a moment that made me truly realize he was so confused and unaware of his mistake. A moment that made me realize my dad probably needed me more than I needed him. I felt as if our relationship had started to shift.

Then there was the day I arrived at the house, and he was at the door to greet me with a smile and a hello. I took off my coat, and he took it from me to hang it in the closet. He paused, handed me a hanger, and said, "Here, can you do it? I don't remember how." My heart felt as if it had stopped. I froze in a bit of shock. My smile faded as I stared at him and his honest confession. This man had cut into people's bodies with such precision and skill to save their lives, and now he couldn't even use a hanger. It was mind-blowing. It was disturbing. It was sad. It was just another reminder of the stark reality of my father's life and how it was changing. When I would see my dad have a moment of lucidity and kindness, such as a greeting from him as I arrived, it felt right, as if the world was okay again. When moments like the hanger situation happened, it felt like a loud, blaring, unexpected noise that jars you out of a comfortable state of quiet or concentration. It was also somewhat inspiring that he admitted it and asked for help. I was impressed and proud of his humility. I responded that particular day by taking the hanger from him and hanging my own coat. There were times I would have pushed him to try and said, "Oh, come on, Dad. Just try to see if you can do it." There had been times when he didn't want to remove his shoes and just sat in his chair, and I said, "Dad? Can you take your shoes off? I know you can." He always obliged me and took them off without incident. That day, I just gave in and took the hanger from him. I knew his disease was really taking its toll if he was openly admitting a lost skill. He had never told me before that he couldn't do something. I respected the fact he said he couldn't do it, and I wasn't going to argue or make him prove himself.

I had to learn to balance dignity with assistance for someone who had never needed my help. It was for someone who wasn't learning a new skill, but was instead trying to remember an old one. My father could no longer help me in the ways he had in the past, and that was something I had to learn to accept. I hated the way it made me feel a bit selfish that I just wanted my dad to be my dad and take care of me. My expectations of our future together had to be adjusted. I had to show respect and sensitivity to someone who had already lived an entire life and was struggling to continue to maintain dignity. I wanted to treat him how I would want to be treated. He was still a human with thoughts and feelings. He was still my dad.

10

When I was around four or five years old, we would pile into my mom's pea green Fiat and drive fifteen minutes through the city of Burlington, Vermont. The water tower with the big red top that reminded me of my mother's Avon lipstick that she had never worn but sat in a bathroom drawer, would come into view, and I knew we had arrived. The hospital campus was sprawling, and my dad's office was in the same building as his research lab. It always had a smell of what my young mind imagined was dead mice, or at least some sort of chemical that made the air smell musty and thick. It was the smell I came to anticipate with any hospital. I loved visiting my dad at work because his secretary always let us pick from a mug of Tootsie Roll lollipops. The lollipops looked like a collection of colorful balloons, as I reached in to choose a flavor. The smell of the lollipop replaced the smell of the office, and I savored the crunchiness and the chewy middle. My dad's office had a large poster of Albert Einstein, and it was like visiting a museum. The piles of papers, books, breakable artwork, or gifts from patients, along with family photographs, lined the shelves and his desk. Every time we visited, things seemed new and interesting, and other than my lollipop, the office had a "look but don't touch" rule.

I never saw any patients or hospital beds during my visits. I did not fear walking those halls or fear the hospital. I was not conditioned to be afraid of the medical world. If we saw my dad, it was for a brief moment between patients or surgeries, and he would breeze by in his white coat and full head of thick black hair. For a short time, we would enter his world away from home, away from us. We were visitors. We didn't walk the halls *with* him. We waited for him to come to us.

***

It had been a year since my father's initial dementia diagnosis. The hospital that my father was now visiting as the patient smelled of disinfectant as my father, mother, and I walked the halls to my father's radiology appointment. The behemoth Ivy League affiliated hospital was nestled between the mountains in New Hampshire about a half-hour drive from my parents' home. It was often referred to as the "Hitchcock Hotel" by so many locals who had resided near it or visited a patient, a nickname using the later part of the hospital's full name. The main entrance looked more like a mall or a hotel foyer, and the floors were surprisingly carpeted. A hospital with carpeting seemed like an oxymoron to me. However, it was welcoming, and if for not the signs and posters, I may have questioned if I was even at a place that provided medical care.

When I first told Denis that my dad was having a PET scan, his immediate response was, "I can take the day off—whatever you need." I was so relieved. I didn't have to ask twice. I tried to be careful with how much time I asked Denis to take off, as he was the sole income earner in our house. I had to delicately balance needing him to cover me in my "job" at home. He was always willing, but I felt guilty ever making him miss work. I tried to be careful with how much time I "required" of him. I worried that if I asked too often or for too many hours, it could jeopardize his position at his company, where he prided himself for hardly ever missing a day. We had decided early on I would stay home with any children we would eventually have. We were both raised by stay-at-home moms, and that had been a dream of mine. I always wanted children, but once I had them and I quit my paying job, the real work started. I felt as if my end of the bargain was to hold the fort down at home, but as we had more children, I felt that I had to almost ration the time I needed from Denis. If I got sick and couldn't care for the kids on any given day, I would need him to stay home. When I added in my parents, it rationed my time even more. I knew it was a somewhat irrational feeling, but not working made me feel that my time was more expendable. I noticed that feeling with a lot of my other stay-at-home-mom friends as well—we felt the burden of the home. I know Denis could feel my stress, as he was often the one I took it out on, whether I was a ball of tears when he arrived home or got snappy on the phone during the day and abruptly hung up on him. We had been together for sixteen years at that point, and we both knew life was getting harder, but our marriage weathered the storm. Denis never lost his cool with me. It just wasn't his character. He got quiet and gave me my space, but he never shouted or got angry. My children got excited if they knew Denis was taking the day off to spend with them, as he always had something brewing in his mind to do with them. He would plan a trip to visit a local farm or museum.

Depending on the season, he would take them fishing, hiking, on a long bike ride, or sledding. Denis loved my father, and he knew what it felt like to see your parents battle an illness, as both of his were cancer survivors many years before. Managing this balance of caring for my parents while taking care of three children, especially Henry, who was barely two years old, began to make me feel as if I was in a tug of war with my own heart. I wanted to be in both places at once, all the time. I wanted to be there for everyone and not miss anything.

Just a few weeks before my father's PET scan, Jacob had an evening concert at his school, and he played the saxophone as part of the fourth-grade band. My parents had planned to get a ride down from a hired driver, come to the concert, and then head home. An hour before the concert, my mother called me with guilt, saying, "I can't believe I did this, but I scheduled the ride for the wrong day. We won't be able to make it. I feel so bad. I am so sorry." My heart hurt for my mother who sounded so sad on the phone and mostly for Jacob. She wasn't a fan of driving at night anymore, especially on a highway, so I knew their only option to come down at that point was if she drove, and that wasn't going to happen. Jacob was so upset when I broke the news to him, as we put on our coats to leave.

"What? What do you mean? Why can't Papa just drive GG down?" he said, holding back his tears referencing the loving names for his grandparents.

"Because he can't. I am sorry," I said solemnly. My children still hadn't been told what was going on with my father. They were young, and dementia was a difficult disease to explain to a child.

"But why?" Jacob kept badgering.

I kept responding, "He just can't! He can't drive anymore!" I finally broke into tears and shouted so he would stop asking. My heart was heavy, my head hurt, and it just wasn't fair. I knew I had to eventually tell Jacob what was going on, and maybe the PET scan would help explain further, so I could do that.

The PET scan, a more thorough diagnostic imaging test of his brain, was required to clarify his diagnosis for Medicare requirements. The test was performed similarly to an MRI. He agreed to the test. The test required minimal, if not zero, mental effort on his part, so I did wonder if this is why he agreed to it, rather than the intense neurological testing he declined a year before. I knew my mother didn't want to, or really shouldn't have to, navigate these appointments alone. I felt helpless in so many other ways for my father and his diagnosis, but I knew I could be with them and offer support in the form of company and a second set of ears. I also wanted to hear firsthand what a doctor said, so my mother didn't feel as if she had to remember everything all by herself in an already stressful time.

It was four days before Christmas, and the three of us walked the halls together wearing our boots and thick winter coats. We trudged along. My father kept pace with me. My mother often stopped and adjusted her purse or the bag she carried. Dad and I then stopped, looked back, and waited. My mother was carrying a brown paper bag with handles that contained a few boxes of chocolates.

"Mom, who are these for?" I asked, eyeing the scrumptious treats when I arrived at their house earlier that day.

"Oh, the secretaries at the hospital. It's Christmas, and everyone needs a little chocolate in their lives," my mother responded with a chuckle. Even in her time of struggle, my mother wanted to give back, to appreciate the people on the other side of the desk. Her generosity never ceased, as long as I had known her. My mother spent the first few years of their marriage working as a medical secretary until she had her first child, my sister, Amy. She was always giving of her time, and later in life, as the wife of the chairman of surgery, she embraced the spouses of the residents under my father's tutelage every year with a luncheon. Both of my parents always remembered what it was like to just be starting out in a career and always gave back to places and people that supported them along the way. My mother loved to give gifts as her way of saying "thank you" or "I'm thinking of you." If a basket showed up at my house full of treats, fruit, or crackers and cheese, I knew it was from my mother before I even read the card. It was just who she was—generous and thoughtful.

"I need a little chocolate in my life too!" I responded with my usual attempt at humor. We both laughed. Comedy was my go-to to diffuse the nerves she and I were both feeling for the appointment that day. Humor was always what I reverted to when I felt the most helpless.

My mother and I appeared more nervous than my father, who walked the halls calmly with a blank look on his face. I was anxious for what the PET scan may reveal. My father was quiet for the most part, following our lead and not asking questions. He either was nervous and didn't show it, couldn't remember why we were there, or felt at ease in the hospital setting where he had spent more than half his life. It's possible it was a combination of all three.

75

Either way, he didn't give up the way he felt, which wasn't anything new for him. I didn't ask if he was nervous. I didn't want to put any of my own thoughts in his head.

We walked to the desk in Radiology, and my mother spoke for my father, checking him in, as I stood back but listened. The secretary asked my father his last name and birth date. He got the last name out and correct, but the birth date was more of a struggle. My mother tersely answered for him, following it up with, "He doesn't know it." *Sigh.* I turned and looked at my father. He kept staring ahead. No expression.

Then he was asked to sign his name. My face grew hot with embarrassment for him. My mother again responded, "He can't sign his name anymore."

The secretary said, "That's okay. Can he draw an X?"

My father reached for the pen and signed something that resembled an X. My mother then handed over the power of attorney and health proxy paperwork she had gathered and signed prior to this appointment. She was officially in charge of my dad now. At that point, for my father, it was a necessary step to take to ensure someone made appropriate decisions for him. Witnessing that event was just another small punch to the gut for me. I felt sad and embarrassed for my father. Luckily, he didn't seem to mind, and he certainly didn't make any comment to me about it. We just turned and walked away.

We sat down to wait, and my mother had to use the restroom, so she left the room. The waiting room was crowded, and Dad and I found seats across from one other. He held the brown paper bag on his lap that was now empty. He sat next to a young man and woman, presumably the parents of the small child who sat on the man's lap. My dad looked and smiled at the child. As the child turned his head, I saw a large scar on it, and my breath caught in my throat out of surprise and then sadness. *That poor child. His poor parents.* My dad just sat there smiling and making a funny face at the child, trying to make him laugh. I know he could see the scar too. There was no way anyone could miss seeing it.

Other than my own children, I never witnessed my father interact with other children. It was sweet, it was innocent, and I remembered he spent so much of his career treating pediatric patients. Sick ones. Hurt Ones. Ones who looked different than others. Children who were disfigured by accidents and sometimes abuse. These children had scars that my father worked to heal and nurture, trying to restore their original look, but it never was the same. He often was called upon to testify in court cases and became an expert witness for many others, recounting over and over again what he had seen, how he interpreted the injuries, and what they could indicate. He was used to seeing traumatic, disturbing, and "hard to look at" things. This must have felt no different. His compassion was shining in that moment, and I felt proud. It was a little peek into my dad, the doctor and the human. He may not have remembered his own birth date, but his heart remembered how to be kind, how to show compassion.

They called his name. He was next. I stood up and ran to the radiology tech first and asked if my mother and I could come too. I quickly reminded him that my father had dementia. He said, "Of course. There is a small waiting room for family outside the scan." I was relieved I didn't have to convince him of our necessity to be with my dad, the need to stay by his side.

We all made the walk down the long dimly lit corridor. We were in the basement of the hospital. It was dark, with no natural light, no windows. Only the sound of our footsteps echoed throughout the hall. The basement of any hospital always freaked me out. I knew what else resided down there too—the morgue.

My father walked behind the tech, and my mother

and I followed. I watched my father walk. He was small to me, a bit hunched, wearing regular clothes, rather than a doctor's coat as he had in the past, and he seemed old. His gray hair was thinning, and his walk was slower and more shuffled than in the past. For some reason, we all walked single file. He was following, rather than leading, in the hospital. He was the one having a procedure done, rather than the other way around. I tried hard not to cry, as I grasped this contradiction. My father, the doctor, now the patient, was a difficult concept for me. He went into the scan, and my mother and I sat next to each other. She let out a big sigh and said, "Andrea, I know you will think this is ridiculous, but I want you to write your father's obituary."

"Mom, oh my God. Seriously? He isn't dying!" *Yet.* I was angry and a bit annoyed she was already burying him. She began to cry, and I did too. She wasn't wrong. My father was dying, but his diagnosis did not have an end date. Of course, I would write it one day for my mother as she requested, but saying yes right then and there felt like a betrayal to my father. I wasn't ready to admit, accept, or attempt to summarize my father's life for a newspaper column. I had barely accepted his illness a year after we first found out. If I wrote it then, before we knew more, before he was really debilitated, I felt as if I would be jinxing him. What if he miraculously recovered? I knew, logically, that was almost impossible, but if I wrote his obituary too soon, what if it meant I sealed his fate? His story wasn't finished. His time wasn't over, and I wasn't ready to write an obituary that felt like a final goodbye.

My father returned to us seemingly unfazed and said, "What's for lunch? I'm hungry." He was serious but had a little grin.

The tech looked at my mother upon their return from the scan, but I had missed it. Years later, my mother ended up telling me the tech had given her the "I'm so sorry" look. She already knew, at that moment, the news wasn't good. We headed home, and my mother sent my father and me out to run last-minute errands for Christmas. My mother got a call from the neurologist approximately two hours after the PET scan, while my father and I were out. The scan revealed a fate that brought my mother to tears, and then a state of quiet shock, after the doctor shared the results. My mother kept this news to herself while she processed it. She told my father two days later and the rest of us on Christmas Eve.

11

---◆◆◆---

Christmas as a child was a time of magic and mystery. It was as if my mother waved a wand, and our house came alive with Christmas decorations and the smell of her walnut snowball cookies lined up in tins to give away. She truly brought the enchantment of Christmas with her quiet enthusiasm and warmth. Our Christmas presents only were brought up and placed under the tree on Christmas Eve, after returning from evening mass. It was a real surprise to wake up on Christmas morning to all the gifts under the tree and the one unwrapped present that Santa had delivered. Our Christmas tree was always real but not picked out and bought until the week (or less) before Christmas. My father had seen too many burn patients arrive to him after their trees dried out and caught fire from being up for too long. It was always a family joke that the tree came in right before

Christmas and was tossed the day after. My mother made sure to make up for our lack of time with a Christmas tree with all of the other decorations and magic she created; she loved Christmas, and in turn, we all did too. My father typically had the camera ready to snap some photos of our Christmas morning. When we were little, we were the stars of the photos, opening our gifts, showing off our "wares," smiling big and proud. As we grew, we often grabbed the camera and took pictures of my parents opening their gifts too. My father usually got a lot of clothes for Christmas, and to be funny, he would put them all on at once and we would take his picture to mark the moment in time. It was a glimpse into his silly side. As teenagers, we forced smiles or tried to hide our acne-ridden faces from the camera. Christmas morning had a different excitement by then, but we were together, and that's what mattered.

***

On Christmas Eve, three days after my father's PET scan, my mother wanted to host all of us at their house for dinner. Amy and her husband, Steve, were visiting, and Liza had come up for a few days. When we arrived, the kids ran ahead and began distracting their aunts with hugs and kisses and pleas of, "Play with me!" Denis and I hung up all the coats and arranged the boots that were left in a pile, so no one would trip. Eventually, I made my way to the kitchen where I found my parents. My mother turned around, and after our greeting of hugs, she said to my dad, "Well, Richard, do you want me to tell her, or do you want to?"

I froze. *Tell me what?*

My dad sort of smiled, shrugged his shoulders, grabbed the counter with both hands, and said, "Well, it's Alzheimer's."

I quickly turned to my mother and back to my father and gasped, "Oh, Dad." My voice cracked, and my eyes welled with tears. I looked at him and tilted my head to show my deep concern. He just stood there. I reached for him, and we hugged. I cried. I knew I couldn't deny it anymore if my father was admitting his diagnosis. To hear him say those words was a moment that felt like slow motion. The world spun around us, but the conversation in that kitchen stopped in time. It felt final and official coming from him. *How do we go on from here? What do we do? How should I act? What should I say?* Instead, my father filled the silence. Finally, I pulled away, wiping at my eyes, and he said matter-of-factly, but with a grin, "Well, something was eventually going to get me."

My mother sniffled at this. I was not surprised he said this. He never wanted sympathy or for us to be upset, especially by something that was his own health issue. He was still trying to be positive; he didn't blame or curse or yell or show anger. I know his disease was already afflicting him, maybe dulling his emotions, but he was just matter of fact and, again, completely right. Yes, something was eventually going to get him. It's going to get everyone single one of us, but my reply that day was simple and tearful, "But, Dad, you are so young."

His time would surely be cut short. *Our* time.

Alzheimer's was different than dementia. I came to understand that dementia is an umbrella, and Alzheimer's sits under it as a more specific form. It affects speech, memory, and physical and mental capabilities. It is a terminal illness with currently no cure. It was a more specific diagnosis, and with it came a tighter possible timeline for my father. It was a more definitive prognosis. The neurologist told my mother, just days before during their phone call, at best, at most, he had ten years left, and that was being generous with time.

On Christmas Eve day, and just shy of his sixty-ninth birthday, my father accepted his fate with grace and even a little humor while the rest of us cried. I found my sisters a few minutes later and whispered, "Did you know?" Amy nodded and said my mother had told her earlier that day. I felt stunned and left behind. I had gone on that whole day not knowing, while my sisters and my parents suffered in this bubble without me. I had walked through the door earlier all loud and excited for the holiday, while they harbored this information. I felt like an outsider. I wished my mother had told me at the same time she told them. Then I realized maybe she was protecting me and allowed me to enjoy that Christmas Eve with my children, blissfully unaware. I forgave her for this and thanked her for that "gift" of time, for the "gift" of not knowing until I was in person, to learn the information straight from the patient himself.

Later that evening, back in the kitchen, long after the sun had set, the steam from the pot rose to warm my face. We were making my paternal grandmother's famous tortellini soup. Raised as a French-Canadian, she married a full-blooded Italian and adopted most of his culture's food customs. She made handmade tortellini with her church friends and always made a soup with the tortellini, one that became a family staple, one that my mother also took on as her daughter-in-law. Rather than eat a salad before our main course, tortellini soup served as our appetizer at most holiday meals. Christmas Eve dinner also arrived in this same manner that night. The memory and tradition of the soup comforted me, as I stared into the pot standing side by side with my mother, as we quietly sighed and sniffled. This soup tradition was not the only thing my grandmother passed down. My father unfortunately had also inherited the awful disease that afflicted her and took her life merely three-and-a-half years before.

The song "When We Were Young" by Adele was playing on the CD player right behind where my father sat at the dining room table. I glanced to my left and saw him in the dark room awaiting his mother's soup that was now my mother's soup. He was a bit hunched over, sitting alone, patiently, quietly. Soon the room filled with talking and laughing and shouts of, "Who needs a glass of wine?" from my sisters, as they made their way into the kitchen. When Adele sang, my throat tightened, and I blinked back a tear. Adele was right. I needed to take pictures before things started to change too much, before my family changed and became unrecognizable to my dad.

The next day, on Christmas, my sisters and parents drove down to my home, and we celebrated the holiday. Adele's song still rang in my ears, and I realized we hadn't taken any pictures of us as a family since my sister Amy's wedding two years before, so I gathered us all on the couch and took out the selfie stick to photograph our group of ten. We had doubled in size from our original number over the last thirteen years. It took a few takes, a few bribes, and a lot of hollers to "Stop! Just smile!" but we managed to all be looking forward and even smile for one last picture as a family. I think we had more fun taking the picture as a family than opening any presents that day. We laughed, and we felt each other's warmth. We all sat huddled on one couch, all ten of us. It was something we didn't normally do as a family—be so close physically. I think we all needed to feel each other's energy that day. It was our version of a family group hug. I continued to take pictures throughout the day. It was important to document this time in our life. Good or bad, this was our family. This was a moment in time we would never get back. It was my turn to be behind the camera, to make sure we had something to look at when time marched on and changed all of us. My dad was wearing a beautiful sweater my mother and him had purchased on a recent trip to Scotland, a trip where he was honored with an international award as a surgeon. His smile was genuine. We could see his eyes were even smiling. The man was told only two days ago he had Alzheimer's, yet he was smiling. He was with his family and celebrating Christmas. To some this was normal, a tradition, but to have my dad home and with us all day was our Christmas miracle. His only thoughts, after my mother delivered the news to him after the PET scan, were that he wanted to spend his remaining days in the home they had built and with his family and wife of forty-four years. My father's bucket list consisted only of being with his loved ones. A simple request. Simple joys would be important for all of us. Recognizing them would be key. Documenting them would be just as important. Memories were still meant to be created, not lost entirely.

12

---◆—◆—◆>——

Seven months after my father's Alzheimer's diagnosis, and a year and a half into his dementia, we went to the ocean. My mother had planned a four-day trip for all ten of us to a hotel and spa on the Maine coast. She wanted her children and grandchildren all together for a few days. It was a time for us to be together, but it was also to celebrate my parents' forty-fifth wedding anniversary. My mother knew my father most likely wouldn't remember or even understand what it meant to have an anniversary anymore. I think she wanted to celebrate the family my father and her had created. The life, or *lives*, they had made, literally. Sadly, it was also a time for her to get a break. It was a place she felt at peace, and the ocean air and sound of the waves was a medicine for the heart and soul that couldn't be found in any pharmacy or doctor's office. Four years before this trip, my sisters, my mother, and I had come to the same hotel. We had come to celebrate my thirty-fifth and Liza's thirtieth birthdays. It was a relaxing trip spent sunning at the pool and dining the down-town, in between shopping in the boutique shops that lined the street. We had massages and pedicures and enjoyed the company of each other, as adult women, with our matriarch. I spent the days missing my children, happy I had the break, and deciding if I was ready to add to my brood. I asked my mother on the trip, "Should I have a third child? Do you think I can handle another one?" She told me only I could truly know the answer to that. She had three, so I figured I could too. I felt as if I needed one more to complete our family. I didn't want to live with a life of regret, and I knew that as I aged, the decision would eventually be made for me. My father retired six weeks later, and I decided to consider trying to get pregnant again. Amy got married the next year, and I was pregnant with Henry at her wedding. The trip with my mother and sisters was the last one we took as a foursome, before our family went from a group of eight to ten.

The nine of us sat at the picnic tables overlooking the ocean, licking our ice cream off of plastic spoons. The kids raced to finish their ice cream cones before the hot July sun melted them away into a soupy mess. My mother had stayed back in her room to get some time to herself. It was time spent not having to constantly worry about my father and tend to all of his needs on her own. It was a break from the constant watching over and assisting that she was no longer used to, since she hadn't had small children in over thirty-five years. She often commented that she felt as if she was losing herself in always caring for my father. It was a familiar feeling, and as a parent with small children, I understood her situation. It can feel as if you forget who *you* are and what *you* enjoy doing, as your time is almost fully devoted to caring for someone else. She, unfortunately, had the added layer of losing her best friend and partner, with my father's decline and his inability to communicate and function as he had before Alzheimer's. I had been with Denis for eighteen years at that point, and he was my best friend and partner as well. I couldn't imagine losing him to a disease like Alzheimer's, as my mother was losing my father. I couldn't imagine having the one person I shared my deepest feelings with, my life, my home, my children, my love, and my future, just slowly slip away from me. Watching my mother lose her connection with my father made me want to cherish my time with Denis even more. Life wasn't perfect or all roses, but I often looked at Denis and realized I could lose him, too, at any time for any reason like an accident or medical event, and that scared me. I was losing my father, but I still had Denis. I still had my rock. My mother was losing hers, and I could see her wilting from it. My sisters and I recognized this fact and tried to take Dad for walks or to get something to eat to ease my mother's responsibility. My father finished his ice cream and seemed itching to get back to my mother. He stood up and said something like, "Probably should get back."

His attachment had grown even more obvious. He was so dependent on her. It was so hard to watch a man like my father not be independent in his tasks or able to make even simple decisions, like what flavor of ice cream he wanted. It was hard enough to worry about my own children, but now I had to manage my father, as well, if we were out in public. When I was out with my children, I had a list of responsibilities that fell to me: their safety, their basic needs, their desires, and their behavior. Sometimes just their safety was enough to monopolize my thoughts, as we crossed a busy road or sat by the ocean. When I added in my concerns for my father, it felt as if I had to expand my web of responsibilities, as he had entered that group of people who needed my care. My sisters gladly stepped in and took Dad under their wing as their responsibility, but I think, being a mother, I felt the most responsible for him; at least that's what I decided to put on myself. At the same time, I was relieved they didn't have the same responsibility of children to take away from them caring for Dad on that trip. I was happy they could step in, but I continued to put pressure on myself to keep an eye on him. I was used to looking out for people who couldn't look out for themselves. I watched him closely for cues to see if he was confused or wanted to use the bathroom. I felt constantly on high alert. We sat at the pool in the warm sun while the kids swam. I normally would have closed my eyes and taken in the delicious warmth and Vitamin D and let Denis watch the kids. Instead, I sat staring at my dad. At times, I felt as if I was drowning from responsibility. I worried about what *could* happen, and I had trouble just living in the moment. It was a personality trait I had mastered in my life at that point, often to my disadvantage. I worried about everything and everyone. Denis sometimes commented, "It's okay, Drea. You don't need to worry so much." I usually agreed but silently disagreed, thinking, *Who will if I don't?* Part of why Denis and I make a great team is that I worry enough for the both of us. In most situations of physical challenge (skiing, hiking, swimming at a rivers edge), he allows the kids to take risks and build their confidence. I sit off to the side, shaking my head, usually mumbling or even shouting, "Please don't get hurt! That looks dangerous!" I know it drives Denis crazy that I am so anxious, but more than once they needed that first aid kit I had brought along on any given excursion.

The hotel sat on a cliff over the ocean, and that's exactly how life felt at times. We were sitting on the edge of something deep, mysterious, and sometimes unknown. My father's illness was like the tide. It ebbed and flowed. Some days, he was so lucid, and other days, he was like a lost child needing his hand held while we walked. My mother was treading water. She was my father's life preserver, while trying to maintain her own buoyancy. She needed a life boat to come rescue her. She made small comments like, "I never have time for myself anymore," or, "He follows me everywhere; I just need a few minutes to breathe." That trip was my mother's respite.

My mother expressed interest in attending a sound healing session at the spa. She asked if any of us wanted to go with her. I had always been willing to get in touch with my spiritual side and try new things, so I agreed to go. We sat in the room listening to the bowls and tuning forks and the woman asked us what our intentions were for being there. My mother could have launched into a whole rant about my father's Alzheimer's and how it was slowly eating away at their marriage and his personality, and life, but all she said was, "I am looking to find some inner peace." She just needed to breathe and to close her eyes and set aside her concerns and responsibilities for an hour. I wanted the same for myself. I answered similarly. Some days, my mother and I connected on our deep feeling of responsibility for everyone around us. She knew my children, some days, felt like an albatross around my neck, as much as I loved them, and I knew now that my father felt the same to her. The constant care and worry and meeting of needs for a man who used to be independent and successful were overwhelming and new for her. Most of all, she missed her husband. Their relationship wasn't the same anymore, as my father changed and slipped inside a world of quiet and confusion. It had gone from husband and wife to man and his caregiver. She was grieving the loss of a man who still shared a bed with her, but not the same marriage.

The last night of our trip, my mother had made a reservation for a private room at the hotel restaurant to celebrate. The floor-to-ceiling windows on one side of the room sat right over the ocean. The adults all had a glass of champagne and toasted my parents. In the past, my dad would have given a small speech, most likely highlighting how wonderful our family was and how special it was to be together, in his usual eloquent words. That time, I think he could tell we hoped he would say *something*, so he did his best. He raised his glass and said, "This is a group of good people." He smiled. He took a sip of his champagne and put his glass down. He looked at all of us as if to say, "Your turn now." That was it. It was all he could manage, and it made me feel sad because he was right, yet I wanted more from him. I wanted him to start talking and never stop. As a child, I would ask my dad about things that I wondered about, like, "What makes a plane take off? How did that work?" and my father would launch into a twenty-minute monologue explaining the physics of flight. I would then regret my question, as my mind wandered, and I tuned out his big, scientific words. I would have given anything that day to hear my dad just go off on some tangent. I looked at my sisters, and they sort of did a quick smile and nod while also fighting back tears. I knew we were all thinking the same thing. We missed Old Dad. At least he tried. It was sweet and thoughtful, but I highly doubt it was what my mother was hoping for after forty-five years of marriage.

I stared at Denis intently. I figured my mother would

have a hard time speaking, as she would have felt too emotional to say what she wanted. My mother was one to write her thoughts down instead, usually in a card. I looked to Denis who often led our family in a short prayer before a meal at home. He caught wind of my expectation that day and did say a few words and congratulated my parents. It helped to diffuse the unfinished feeling my father had left with his abrupt toast.

While waiting for our meal, my mother stood behind my father, leaning over him with her hands on his shoulders, and I snapped a photograph of them. We had taken a similar photo when we celebrated their thirtieth wedding anniversary. So much had changed in those fifteen years, aside from the obvious physical changes that come with age. What hadn't changed was my mother's support for my father, the woman behind the man. It reminded me of what she always said about him and his success in life: "Behind every successful man is a supportive woman." In my parents' relationship, this was the absolute truth. My father smiled but looked distant. The look in his eyes wasn't the same anymore. It was a vacant look, almost glazed over and unfocused, as if his mind was completely somewhere else. Lost at sea.

Halfway through the meal my daughter, Hannah,

who was almost six, complained she wasn't feeling well. She said she felt sick to her stomach. My mind replayed what she had eaten throughout the day, and as any mother would do, I panicked at the thought of the stomach bug striking her and the rest of the family—a vacation nightmare. My sister, Amy, piped up right away and said, "I'll take her to the bathroom." I was grateful she responded and offered. I normally would have taken Hannah myself, but Amy was willing, and I was relaxed from the glass of champagne that was running through me. Amy didn't have children and most likely wouldn't, so I knew these offers were well intentioned, and I felt it was her way of saying, "I know you need a break. Let me."

I said, "Okay, but text me if she isn't okay." Amy and Hannah didn't return to dinner, but when we were all finished with dinner and left, I found them sitting in the lounge outside the restaurant. Hannah was feeling better. She hadn't gotten sick. *How odd,* I thought. I started to rack my brain. Why would she feel better once she left the restaurant? Was it a bad smell? Then I started to put two and two together and realized it.

"Hannah, was the water making you sick? The ocean?" The ocean view in the room sat over the water like a boat floating. There was no ground below to be seen.

"I think so," she said. Hannah had also been getting carsick lately and wasn't able to read whenever we drove anywhere, since she said it made her feel sick to her stomach. She was getting seasick from the restaurant. On land. Once she left the restaurant, she felt better. Hannah just needed to leave to feel better, to get her sea legs back. She needed someone to walk with her, tell her to take some deep breaths, and get her bearings. To change her focus.

Just like Hannah, my mother needed to get her sea legs back, ironically *at* the ocean. She needed to leave her element, to leave what was throwing her off balance. She needed to re-center and focus. She needed someone to help, to step in and walk with her. My father had always been her partner, her support, the one to walk with her and hold her up. Life had changed. As a family, you need to look out for each other, recognize when someone needs you, and work together as a team to send out the lifeboat when someone is sinking.

13

---◆--◆--◆---

The month after our trip to the ocean, on a muggy August day, we moved into a new home. Our family had outgrown the house and yard in the neighboring town, and though we were leaving the school system and neighbors, I wasn't leaving my friends. We would be living about twenty minutes from each other, still see each other, and talk as often as we did before. I needed my friends close by, the ones who knew me and what I was going through. I had shared my father's news with them right away, after my mother had told me back on that November day. We were the kind of girlfriends who watched each other's kids in an emergency, met for drinks at the restaurant down the road, met at the playground for play dates, and did weekend getaways with just us girls. Our kids were friends, and we walked the motherhood path together.

We moved about ten minutes closer to my parents, so it was a win-win situation. I felt my friends were my main support, outside of my family, and to have them close by was important. I knew moving would open up a world of new people in our lives, and as much as it excited me, it also scared me to have to essentially start over. I would have to build friendships from "scratch" and build trust in others. I was in the process of learning to trust myself and my decisions, especially big ones, without my dad's opinion. We purchased the new home without my dad's guidance, something I had depended on in the past. It was our third home, and with the other two, my dad had given his opinion, asked me pointed questions about the status of the roof or basement, and even had attended the inspection on my second home. Denis and I made this decision together, and it felt good to trust ourselves and know we could do it all on our own. Though I missed my dad's opinion and advice, I realized I didn't need his approval to be successful. What is it about losing our parents that makes us finally feel like adults?

A few days after moving in, my new neighbor, Leigh, and her daughter came down our driveway with huge smiles, carrying a plant as a gift to welcome us to the neighborhood. We began chatting, and she asked what I did for work. I replied with my standard issue response of, "I stay home with the kids," and then I felt compelled to say, "But I really want to be a nurse someday if I can do it."

"Why not now?" Leigh asked with energy and confidence.

"Um, oh, I just don't have the time," I said and then, for some reason, I went further. I don't know why, on that day, I decided to share my father's diagnosis, but something came over me, and I continued. "Right now, I am splitting my time between my kids and my parents. My dad has Alzheimer's."

Right away, she replied, "Oh, I am so sorry to hear that. My husband's father had that too. He died a few years ago from it, very young." She went on to share a bit of his story and that his mother actually ran a bed and breakfast that also welcomed caregivers of dementia patients to come for respite. If that wasn't a sure sign from God that we had moved to the right place, I didn't know what was. That quickly filled my bucket labeled "Everything happens for a reason." I was meant to meet her and her husband, Rob. My mother was meant to meet his mother and share their stories, and my neighbor had a daughter the same age as Hannah. It was like a gift. I had moved away from my friends, but this new house already felt like home.

The year before we moved, around Henry's first birthday, I decided it was the year I was going to try and go to nursing school. I am not sure if my father's diagnosis or Henry's dance with his health as an infant inspired me to do it then, but I decided, two months after my father's diagnosis, to look into a nursing program. For as long as I could remember, I had always wanted to be a nurse. One day in college, I announced to my roommates that I was going to go to nursing school after we graduated, and they all said, "Good for you. You can do it!" I never went. The science prerequisites scared me off, and finishing a four-year degree had just about tapped me mentally from going on in any further educational pursuits. I settled into a job, my marriage, and then began having children.

After Hannah was born, I spent two years working in an urgent care office as a secretary and quit when I got pregnant with Henry. I worked the Sunday shift and loved every minute of it. It was interesting, exciting, fulfilling, and it only solidified my feelings of wanting to be a nurse. One day, I said to one of the nurses I worked with that I wanted to pursue nursing, and she said I should, "Absolutely do it, and age doesn't matter." Sometimes, after a particular interesting day at work, I called my parents and shared a story with my dad. It felt like a way to bond with him over medical topics. I learned a lot in my two years working there, both clinically and personally. Helping people, especially sick people, made me feel as if I was a little closer to my dad, even if we weren't together. I shared a story with him about a little girl who declined quickly in the waiting room due to a breathing issue and how she had to be sent to the hospital in an ambulance. The mother had come to the window a few times, complaining her daughter was having trouble breathing, even after being triaged by the nurses. At first, I just reminded her of the wait time, but after the third time, she seemed truly frightened by her daughter's breathing. I finally panicked a bit myself at her desperation. I didn't want to question a mother's intuition anymore at that point. I tried to put myself in her shoes. I left the desk to advocate on her behalf to a nurse. "I think this girl really needs to be seen, like now," I said to the nurse who looked at me, and after working together long enough over the months I had been there, she trusted my judgment and jumped into action. My dad said he was proud of me that day for reacting the way I did to push for her, on behalf of the mother, to be seen sooner. He told me children can decline surprisingly quickly and "go down like an airplane that has lost its engines," when their breathing becomes more difficult. He said I did the right thing that day, and I never forgot his words of wisdom about breathing. After that, I was more attuned to watching children as they sat in the waiting room. I loved connecting with my father that way, but more so, I loved that I made him proud. It further enforced my desire to become a nurse.

Once Henry started walking, and Denis and I decided he was our last child, I felt as if it was my time to finally follow my dreams. Looking back, I am not sure if I did it following my father's diagnosis in an attempt to help him, be prepared medically for what was to come, or if it was to actually distract my mind from what was happening with my dad. The day I told my parents I wanted to go to nursing school, they were both caught off guard. My dad was only a few months into his dementia diagnosis, and he didn't seem too keen on me going back to school. My dad walked me to the car that day, and as I got in to leave, he said, "I just know it's a lot of work. For years, I've seen nurses really get stressed out. Give your mom and me time to process this one. I process slower these days." I was sort of angry he said that. *Why couldn't I do it, too*? I thought he would be supportive of me, but I think he knew another side of nursing and didn't want my life to get any more stressful with the three kids.

I said, "Okay, Dad. I get it," quietly, but with a bit of attitude, and I shut the door and drove home. I felt disappointed and hurt that he didn't think I should become a nurse and then I felt more awful that I was mad at a man who had dementia and was trying to guide me in the best way he thought. I think my mom's lack of support stemmed from her not wanting to lose me while she was, at the same time, losing my father. Nursing school would surely consume my entire life if I let it. I could understand where she was coming from, but her lack of support hurt too. My parents were usually supportive of decisions I made in life, so to lack their support in that was somewhat shocking, but as an adult and parent, I tried to look at it from their points of view. I was still hurt and upset by it, but they were thinking of my well-being and mental health, while all I saw was a dream being dashed with their words.

I didn't let my parents' opinions sway me, though. I pushed forward in doing what I wanted to for myself. I had to try. I began my prerequisites and took a medical ethics course first. It was fascinating, eye-opening, and an emotional journey for me so soon after my father's diagnosis. I typed papers while Henry napped or sat at my feet playing with a toy. I spent my weekend days listening to a lecture while Denis took the kids out or kept them occupied. I studied philosophy and, eventually, topics like abortion, euthanasia, and stem cell research in regards to medical ethics. I did well in the class and was proud of the A I earned. Taking a medical ethics class felt like a little peek into my father's career world. I shared my papers with my mother, and she was astounded at the work I had done. I was proving I could do it. I could raise three kids and take a class and still be available to my parents. Once in a while, I tried to ask my father for his opinion on a topic, but I knew his comprehension and communication were getting more challenging for him. It propelled me to want to continue, and, most of all, it kept me from constantly worrying about my dad. I had my studies and my children and my eye on the prize. After the class ended, I eventually lost steam. I put off my next class for two semesters, as the textbook reading requirement and workload seemed more daunting and demanding than the first class. Henry required more of my attention, and I felt as if my time with my dad was getting shorter. My father continued to decline, and I had to decide where I really wanted to put my energy and time. My dreams for the future took a backseat, especially knowing my future could wait, while my father's future was slipping away. When we decided to sell our home and move, that took first priority, and I packed my dreams of nursing school neatly into a box and placed it on a shelf until further notice, unsure when I would reopen it.

My father's diagnosis would one day be motivating for me, but it was also an excuse to slow my life down. Nursing school would have to wait until I could devote more time and commitment to it. I had to decide if that was my true path in life, but that day, telling my neighbor about my father, was meant to happen. It opened a conversation and a vulnerability for both of us that allowed for a connection that I didn't have with other peers. It helped me begin to see that sharing with people outside of my family and with close-knit group of friends could open up more possibilities for support. It wasn't something to be ashamed of or embarrassed about, and it allowed others to share a connection we may have that would have otherwise gone unnoticed. Though I had initially thought the move would close me off from having close relationships with new friends, it actually opened the door, if I let myself become vulnerable. I was learning to trust myself, depend on myself, and realize I didn't need anyone's approval but my own.

14

───◁◆▷───

Summer melted into fall, which blew into winter. I sat in my gown under the blinding and revealing lights and crossed my arms. There was a gentle knock on the door, and my OB/GYN entered the room. I had known her for eleven years at that point, since the day we met at Jacob's birth. I trusted her. She went through my medical history and then to the question I was dreading. "Has anything changed in your family history since I last saw you?" I knew I was going to be honest, that I *had* to be. Not long after my dad was diagnosed with Alzheimer's, I had the life changing thought, *Oh no. He has Alzheimer's. We are related. I could get this too.* So now, coupled with my own dad's diagnosis, I always had that nagging little bug in the back of my brain constantly reminding me. *This could happen to you too.* It was terrifying. Would I wake up one day and forget how to tie my shoes or button my shirt? Would

I lose my gift of gab? Would I become someone who became dependent on someone else to function? Would I need Denis in the way that my father needed my mother?

"Um, yeah. My dad has Alzheimer's. He was diagnosed a year ago, and two years ago with dementia." I choked out the words. I couldn't go on without crying, so I stopped.

She turned away from her laptop and looked at me, "Oh, my God. You poor thing. Here you are sitting under these awful bright lights, half-dressed, and crying. I am so sorry." She handed me some tissues, sat back down, and asked me more about my dad. She was compassionate, thoughtful, and patient.

She finally asked, "Will you get the test that tells you if you carry the gene?"

I hadn't ever considered it, but I quickly replied, "No. I don't want to know what's coming for me."

She nodded her head and said respectfully, "I can understand that." I had answered without much thought but knew that if I had a test that told me I was going to get Alzheimer's, it would be like a dark cloud over my head every day. If I knew it was going to happen, and it was just a matter of time, it would be too much for me to handle. I would be consumed by worry, rather than hope that it might not. I chose hope rather than truth at that point, for myself and my future. And I chose to be proactive.

That was the day I decided to live my life a bit differently. I was going to take better care of myself, lose weight, drink less alcohol, and maybe move up my timeline on the trip to Italy I had been planning for retirement. I had read about some of the possible risk factors, and I wanted to try and minimize them if I could. I started to tell everyone in my life, "I'm going to Italy when I turn forty-five, and Denis and I celebrate our twentieth anniversary. Life is short." If I couldn't cure Alzheimer's, I was going to try and stave it off as best as I could. I was going to do things sooner and not wait. I wanted to take control of the things I could, like my mental and physical health, yet I didn't want to know my fate. I didn't want to go to bed every night wondering if the next morning, I was going to wake up and feel different or forget something. I didn't want to question if today was the day my cognition had entered a new phase because of a gene that dictated my future.

I texted my sisters and told them about my new revelation. I asked how they felt. They both agreed they didn't want to know for themselves either. We all did admit, though, that we now questioned ourselves more.

We were more paranoid about our own mental acuity since my father's diagnosis. I told them I sometimes couldn't remember the word for something, and they admitted the same. Amy was only forty-three, and Liza was thirty-five, so we agreed it was most likely just the stress and overwhelming daily life that kept us from functioning at one hundred percent at all times. I blamed my three kids and loud dog. We sent laughing emojis about my kids and dog but promised to keep an eye on each other. We knew that since both my grandmother and at least three, maybe even four, of her sisters and my dad suffered, that we might be next.

Thank God I had my sisters to deflect to during all of this. They were my saving grace so many times. I didn't feel alone in my thoughts about my dad. I could vent to them without guilt because I knew they wouldn't judge me for my feelings, and even if they did, they never said it. We were experiencing the same loss of the same father, and I was grateful not to be alone on that journey. I knew I could text them any feeling, inappropriate, unfair, mean, or even a sweet dad story, and knew they would respond with what I needed. An "I get it. Totally. Aw," or sometimes, "I know. It's so hard." I will forever be grateful that my parents gave us each other. We needed to be together to get through this. I, of course, could share my feelings with Denis or my mother or a friend, but my sisters and I were often very similar in our feelings toward situations. They knew my father the way I knew my father, and seeing him change affected us all. I wasn't losing a spouse or the love of my life. I was losing my, *our,* father, and only my sisters could understand that. I told my sisters I cried a lot in the car when I was alone, and Amy admitted she cried every night on her way home from work, if she got to thinking too much about my dad. She lived the farthest away, and I know her heart felt pulled in both directions—to move closer to my parents, but also to stay in Illinois. We all kept in constant contact with my mother, usually with a daily text or phone call, even if it was to just say hello. Our moral support for my parents was the most abundant and easy thing we could provide when we couldn't be there physically.

We were a united front, with a common bond and goal to keep my parents' well-being as a focus. Many times, I would send a text to them, hoping for a bigger response than I got. I think I spent more of my days obsessing over my parents than my sisters did. They had careers to distract them, and in the quiet of my home, if my kids were entertained and I had two seconds to think, it was usually to worry about my parents. Amy kept her opinions more to herself unless directly asked, and Liza listened when I just needed to vent. I also was living on the "front lines" more obviously, since I lived close to my parents and frequented them the most.

It's not to say we weren't without fault at times. I knew that sometimes my sisters thought I was overly emotional, too reactive, or passionate, that I cared too much or said too much to my mother about what I felt was best. There were times I was too sensitive and took things too personally. Liza went to visit my parents one weekend and called me on her way home to fill me in on her visit.

"So, when I got there, the caregiver told me Dad's smile, and him getting up to greet me, meant he knew who I was, and she said that because he seemed to react with so much emotion!" my sister said, recounting the caregiver's comment to me.

Oh, great. I immediately responded with jealous venom. "Oh, that's nice. Dad had zero reaction when I visited last week. I guess he doesn't know me now. Good for you!" I spat back. I was angry. I was sad. I was jealous. I was mad that she had rubbed that in my face. Then, I felt guilty that I was mad at her. She was innocent and would never intentionally make me feel bad. Liza wasn't like that;

it would pain her to ever know she had hurt someone's feelings.

"I'm sorry, Dre. I didn't mean it like that. I didn't even think of that," Liza quickly shot back, a sullenness hanging in her voice.

I apologized, too, but still felt wounded. I would get over it, but not right away. I was grieving the loss of Old Dad, and I was jealous. I was jealous that my sisters didn't have to constantly choose between spending time with my parents or their children. I was jealous I didn't have a job outside of my home to distract my thoughts more. Liza put in many long weekends at my parents helping out with my dad. She was the bravest of us. She got right in there and helped change him or bathe him. Maybe it was working in a hospital that made her like that, or maybe she just was a bit stronger emotionally to be able to handle that level of involvement. Either way, I admired her for it. Amy spent a week at a time at my parents' when she came to visit, something that I most surely wouldn't have been able to do, logistically or emotionally. I began to realize my time was limited to only a few hours that I could handle, both emotionally and often logistically due to my children's schedules and other life commitments such as appointments, the dog, or needing to be home to maintain a routine. My involvement was more regular but was for shorter stints since I lived so close. Living within a thirty-minute drive and not being tied to a career allowed me this ability. I talked to my mother daily and attempted to shoulder the emotional burden of her pain and frustration, while trying to balance my own and my children's needs.

My sisters and I sometimes disagreed on how much we should actually involve ourselves with my dad's care. On any given day, one of us might make the statement, "I give up. I can't do this anymore." By "can't do this anymore," we meant worry. Discuss. Try and solve a problem that couldn't be solved. We couldn't cure my father or force my parents to do things we thought were best or better. We couldn't force them to go to Boston for further medical treatment or branch out more in the community that was still somewhat new to them since retirement. We couldn't make them live a life they didn't want to; they were adults and had their own life outside of us. Of course, by the next day, we were back on board, discussing and worrying about my parents. One day, I commented that all we ever talked about was Mom and Dad. Our texts were no longer about our own lives. My sisters wrote back saying, "Wow, you are right." After that, I made an effort to text about myself once in a while, something completely unrelated to Dad or Alzheimer's. I didn't want our only connection to be over my parents. I wanted to make sure we still let each other into other parts of our lives, too. I realized there was time and space for all of our worries, humor, and triumphs to coexist together. Our emotional health was just as important as our physical health. We were learning that it was important to balance all of it, as we walked the journey together.

15

---◆－◆－◆---

The sound of a low motor woke me from my deep sleep. I rolled over and looked at the clock. The time 5:15 A.M. glared back at me in a harsh, blue glow. The motor made rhythmic noises, as it went up and down the driveway. I had high school later that day, or maybe it would be canceled. The snowblower continued back and forth. My father was clearing his path to leave for work. A man and his toys. He woke earlier than his usual 5:30 A.M. time and started the snowblower, waking me, and probably the entire neighborhood, in the process. The sound always annoyed me, while offering comfort at the same time. It was loud and disruptive, but it meant my dad was taking care of us, clearing the way, with the anticipation of what had fallen the night before still to be seen, as I lay warm and content under the covers.

***

My father gave up driving first. We didn't have to beg for his keys or hide them from him. He had hit the garage one day a few months after his diagnosis. It wasn't a big hit, but some of the cedar siding had broken off of a small corner where it looked like a vehicle missed navigating a turn. He told my mother, "That was it." He didn't trust himself to drive anymore. She was relieved. His car sat in the garage for months. Finally, my sister, Amy, and her husband flew out and purchased the car from my parents and drove it the 1,000 miles back to Illinois. It was her little (big) piece of Dad she could maintain in his honor.

Though my parents had only lived in New Hampshire full-time for four years, my father had a shed, basement room, and garage full of tools. He had two tractors and more shovels, rakes, screws, drills, and hammers than Home Depot. He had accumulated them over the years, and when my parents moved, he brought everything with him and continued to add to his supplies. His supplies came in handy many times for a small project, something that needed fixing or building, or just the occasional lost nail or screw that needed replacing. My father grew up working in my grandfather's auto parts store, and I imagined that being surrounded by his own tools gave him a sense of comfort and nostalgia for that time. Maybe being surrounded by endless parts and tools made him feel connected to his own father, while also being prepared for anything.

My dad's hands were always busy in and out of the operating room. These tools assisted in him whatever job came up in the house, garage, or yard that needed his attention. Denis came to depend on my father's supplies, and if we had a project at home and needed something like a table saw or special tool, Denis said, "I bet your dad has one I could borrow." Denis always said "borrow," never "have." He never wanted to take and keep anything of my father's without express permission, and he never wanted to assume that what was my father's would end up being his. He had a lot of respect for my father, and their relationship was one of mutual love and admiration. The summer after Denis and I began dating, he stayed with my family in Illinois during a summer accounting internship. My father and Denis grew close that summer working alongside each other in my parents' yard, doing various tasks on the weekends. Denis growing up on a Vermont dairy farm with a strong French-Canadian background, reminded my father of his mother's family and his own grandparents. My father came to know that Denis was a man of integrity, hard work, and respect. My father observed our relationship grow over the four years we dated, and when my father walked me down the aisle at our wedding and handed me off to Denis, he didn't just hug me and hand me off; he put his arms around the both of us, at the same time, and we had a group hug.

When we bought our new home following my dad's diagnosis, it came with three acres, and Denis knew he would need a tractor to maintain the property. My mother offered for him to buy my father's smaller John Deere. Denis jumped at the chance, and "Janie," the John Deere tractor, as my son Jacob so lovingly named her, found a new home with us. My father didn't say much about the purchase, but I could tell he was happy to see it go to Denis. My husband, being raised on a farm, knew hard work and how to run and care for a tractor. My son was also a tractor enthusiast, so naturally, they embraced this new toy, or *tool,* as my husband and father had corrected me years before.

My mother also asked me to sell my father's larger tractor for her. This John Deere had a backhoe, and my father drove it around their New Hampshire property with a grin while he moved branches or pushed the snow. He gave Jacob rides on it, but my father could no longer remember how to operate it, and it wasn't safe even if he could. Denis drew up the purchase and sales document, and I coordinated the Craigslist ad and sale. The day the man came to purchase it, my father stayed inside. My mother knew he wasn't able to formulate answers to any questions about it and saved him the embarrassment. He didn't complain or act disappointed when it left on a trailer behind a pickup truck. Another joy lost; another freedom given up. My father humbly let his hobbies slip away. Maybe it was apathy, but I like to think it was maturity, grace, and acceptance. He knew his boundaries and was protecting himself and others from the dangers he could encounter. My father came in from changing the oil in his tractor, a few months prior to us selling it, and his hands stunk. I said, "Dad, you stink like gas! You should wash your hands." He looked down and smelled his hands. He couldn't smell them. At all. He washed them a few times, and I smelled them again. They still stunk. "Dad, you can't smell this? It's awful!" I was more concerned with the need to mention it a second time to him.

He just shook his head and muttered, "No, not really."

His sense of smell had been lost for a few years at that point, and my mother assumed it was from his many years in the operating room and the chemicals that floated around him. Except, it was his disease. It was the first sign that we knew, looking back, of his Alzheimer's. A sign that we didn't equate to anything at the time.

I admired the responsibility and maturity behind my mother's decisions to sell or distribute these items. She wasn't trying to pretend it wasn't happening. She may not have liked it, but she did it anyway. Maybe it was her way of coping; maybe it hurt her too much to look at all the things that once brought my father such joy. I know she was sad to see a part of my father leave with each purchase, but she accepted that he would never be the same man he was when he used those tools. I wondered if she thought ahead and didn't want to have to do all of it right after my father died—that it would be too painful then. I tried to think to myself which was worse. Then, while he seemed aware of it happening, or after, when we just had his things left to remind us? Both concepts were painful in their own right, and I let my mother decide which pain she would rather endure. My mother did these things slowly and methodically. She didn't do it all at once and never made a big deal of it. It was a fact of the disease. It was a necessary act.

When Denis and I visited together, my mother would say, "Please, take anything you need. Just take it," referring to any tools or yard items we might need. It pained me to do this. I was cleaning out my dad's life while he sat in a chair and watched it all. I felt as if I was robbing them and taking what wasn't mine, but I also felt that if not us, then who would be better? Denis treated my father's things with gentleness, and that tractor sat in our shed, clean, well-maintained, and loved. The greatest legacy to his tools was to keep them as he would have. To respect their power and use them wisely, appropriately. That my dad's tools were now our tools. That we could keep his memory alive and honored if we used them as he intended, as he would want to do for us, if he still could.

16

Two years into my father's diagnosis, my mother broke down and admitted she needed help with my dad. He required more of her time, all of her time, and she was getting burnt out. They had been attending a Memory Café group, where other people with dementia and Alzheimer's went with their caregivers to participate in a support group. My father told my mother he didn't like going anymore. "I think he gets too overwhelmed with the people and the multiple conversations going on," my mother told me one day, after a group meeting. My father had been getting more anxious in group settings, so this was not a positive outing for him. My mother enjoyed the meetings, as long as no one monopolized the conversation, as some often did. If my father wasn't going to go out, then my mother realized she needed to have someone come to them instead.

My mother, sisters, and I discussed options for caregivers, debating between agencies and private people for hire. We researched online what the area had to offer. I found some people and even placed some ads on a caregiving website. If someone applied for the job and I felt they were well-suited for my parents, I passed along the info to my mother. Amy and Liza found agencies online and called around, seeing what the scope of care was and what methods of payment were accepted. We did a bit of the due diligence, and my mother had the final say if she wanted to move forward with a place or person. She set up some interviews and eventually had to tell my dad what was going to happen. She went over and over it again with him, but it wasn't really sinking in for him. In general, and for lack of a better term, my father needed a babysitter. He needed someone to entertain him, watch out for him, and be with him when my mother couldn't be or when she needed a break. He needed a paid companion. I didn't fault my mother for needing help; if anything, I encouraged it.

"Mom, if you can get a break but still have Dad around and know he's well taken care of, it's the best of both worlds. You should be allowed to enjoy your relationship with Dad and not have it be all about being a caregiver all the time," I told her one day, when she was struggling to accept the fact others may have to care for my dad as well. I think she thought it meant she was a failure as a wife, but I felt she deserved to get a break and just be able to enjoy my father's company, not needing to tend to his every need.

I drove my dad into town one day to get some groceries and tried to approach the subject. "Dad, I heard you will be having someone come and help now."

He was quiet, looking out the window. "Yes. Your mom said that, but why?" I told him we all needed a little help sometimes, that it was okay, and that someone like a nurse was there to help him. He seemed confused and asked me if this person was working for him or with him.

I said, "Sort of both." I tried to be careful in my response. I didn't want to make him feel stupid or embarrassed.

His confusion continued. I finally realized why he was confused once he said, "But I don't do that anymore. It's not my job." So much of talking to my father then was like trying to decode a hidden message. I used to say it was like a constant game of Password. He spoke, but his point wasn't always clear or concise.

When I said nurse, he thought I meant because he was a doctor and that a nurse would be helping him. "Oh no, Dad. You aren't a doctor anymore like that. This person will help you, so you can rest now. It's your time to take a break from that long career."

He agreed and said flatly, while still looking out the window, "Yeah… a break."

I couldn't bear to explain the absolute truth to him. I couldn't bear to tell him that Mom needed time away and that he needed to be watched and entertained, so she could have time to herself. My mother loved my father, but his care was taking its toll on their relationship and my mother's overall health. She was mentally and physically exhausted from doing so much for him every day, including spending hours quizzing him on basics like his letters and numbers. She was trying to keep him sharp mentally, while sacrificing her own rest and downtime.

I helped with some of the interviews, and typically, my father was present as well. It felt uncomfortable talking about his deficits and needs in front of him. He usually remained quiet during the interviews. My mother often referred to him as "not your average Joe." This was her way of describing my father's extreme intellect and that he was still able to "get by" with some things, but overall, he was becoming dependent in many ways. He had forgotten how to use the microwave, for example, so he needed help with that. During one interview, my mother said how much she helped my father and how much she did for him and took care of him. All of a sudden, he chimed in, quietly but with a smile and assurance, "I helped you too." He didn't elaborate, but I made sure to follow it up and try to clarify his statement.

"I think Dad means he helped you with your health and even saved your life once during an allergic reaction." I replied, looking at my dad to see his reaction.

He nodded his head in agreement, and he had a proud look on his face.

"This is true," my mother said, half laughing. I think she enjoyed these little moments of lucidity from my father. I know I did. He was still there. He was listening.

The caregivers started out slowly—a few hours a day, a few days a week. They made his lunch, watched TV with him, took him to his dentist or hair appointments, walked with him around the neighborhood loop, and assisted with bathroom needs and clothing changes. He was happy and, for the most part, enjoyed their company but always had his eye on my mother. If she left the house, he was there to greet her at the door when she arrived home. He worried. My mother commented, a year or so into my dad's diagnosis, that he didn't know her anymore. "He doesn't call me Mary anymore. I don't think he knows my name or who I am to him." I disagreed with her. I think my dad knew who we all were to him but couldn't pronounce our names anymore or possibly remember them exactly.

Then she called me one day in a moment of pure joy. "Your dad was waiting at the door when I got home. He kissed me!" That was the highlight of her month, maybe even her year. He didn't kiss just anyone when they walked into the house.

While my mother got a bit of a reprieve, the caregivers were also my saving grace, all while having the idea of their presence reminding me I wasn't enough. I wasn't the one to care for my dad. I struggled with the idea that it should be me, that I was supposed to be the one to help my parents, but ultimately, I couldn't and didn't necessarily want to be the one. If a caregiver didn't show one day, and I could manage it, I would go up for a few hours. I ran small errands, sorted laundry, and did the dishes. I kept my father company at times, but overall, I wanted my relationship with my dad to be not one of providing his care, but trying to preserve what we had left as a father and a daughter.

As time went on, caregivers came and went as if they were on a conveyor belt, going around and around, dropping off and picking up some along the way. My father was easy to care for, but scheduling and the need for more hours meant a change of caregivers quite often. My mother would send a text to my sisters and me on any given day, announcing that a caregiver had quit or not shown up for a shift. Every time a text came in, my heart would drop; I ached for my parents to have the care they needed and deserved on a regular basis. My mother agreed to interview more agencies and finally found one that seemed to be in line with my parents' needs. My father required more assistance in the bathroom, so this was a prerequisite for his caregivers to be able to help with. The start of a new caregiver was always bumpy. My mother would spend the entire time with them, training them to care for my dad, teaching them about the house and where things were and also to get to know them a bit. If my dad tried to tell a story, my mother was there to fill in the back story or translate his ideas. Eventually, they found dependable and compassionate caregivers who were excellent for my father. If I knew they were there, I could breathe a little easier, and the guilt of it not having to be me lifted off my shoulders, slightly. I often had to remind myself I had three children that I was caring for, that my parents were my family, and I loved them, but they were not my sole responsibility all of the time. That was a hard concept for me to let go of and accept. I am not sure I have ever been able to let go of that concept completely. I will always feel a commitment and responsibility for them, just as I will for my own children, for the rest of my life and theirs. But, I have relieved some of the pressure I put on myself, through the passing of time and beginning to trust other people like the nurses and caregivers.

I made the trip up one day to meet a new caregiver, and I brought Henry along. So much of my visits now were a difficult balancing act of either finding care for my children or bringing them along, and if so, managing their behavior while I tried to have a semblance of a normal visit with my parents. It was exhausting. If I could get in a ten-minute conversation with my mother, without interruption, I was lucky. I had to learn to accept that life wasn't the same anymore. I chose to structure my visits around my father having a caregiver present, so I knew he was cared for, and I could turn my attention to my mother to foster the relationship between her and my children. I knew that was going to be important, as we continued to head down the path of my father's illness. I wanted to make sure I focused on the future and who would be left behind once my father's battle with Alzheimer's ended. The caregivers were strangers to my family but became friends and people we depended on to get us through a scary, unsure, and often stressful time. If my father was to stay in my parent's house for the duration of his illness, the caregivers and any other help was necessary to keep my mother afloat mentally, physically, and emotionally.

17

My dad had an appointment with his neurologist who wanted to see him every six months. He was two and half years into his diagnosis. We rode up north to the "Hitchcock Hotel," aka hospital, and the car was quiet. My mother hired a driver this time, so we didn't have to worry about parking and navigating the vast mother-ship hospital. My mom dozed off, and my dad sat quietly, looking out the window once in a while. I sat next to the driver, trying to keep a conversation going, yet I wasn't truly interested in talking then, either. I was anxious to get through the appointment. I hadn't yet witnessed my father at a neurologist appointment. I wasn't sure how any of it was going to go. Only three years prior, my father had come to this same building with Denis and me to visit a neurologist to rule out a tethered spine for Henry. *Oh, how the tables had turned.*

At that point in his disease, my dad needed help with his seatbelt. I had to unbuckle him and guide him out of the car, while making sure my mother also got out without incident. Her autoimmune disease often rendered her a bit weaker, so I made sure to watch out for her too. It was a slow walk in, but we finally made it. We checked in with the secretary, and my mother did all the talking while Dad and I stood listening. We sat in the waiting room, and I looked around at the other patients and families. Most were older like my dad, one or two were around my age, and I tried to quickly guess why everyone was there. Too many choices. Stroke? Brain tumor? Traumatic brain injury? Alzheimer's? Before I could make up stories for everyone's visits in my head to pass the time, they called my dad, and all three of us walked in together. I was the support for the support system. The backup. I wasn't sure what my father understood or processed anymore. He very well may have been able to listen and understand it all, but without his ability to communicate clearly anymore, it was often a mystery to us what he truly understood. The nurse began to triage my dad in a small little room that was separated from other patients by curtains.

"Do you know your name?" she asked, while typing on a computer at the same time.

"Yes. Richard," my dad responded without a pause.

"And do you know your last name?" she then asked.

"Yes," my dad said shyly. He hesitated. I had a rush of nervousness and embarrassment for my dad. I looked at my mom who finally said, "Richard, what's your last name?"

"It's... It's..." he stammered. Nothing. No name was spoken.

The nurse questioned, "Is it Gamelli?"

"Yes, Gamelli," my dad replied with the insinuation that of course it was! *Duh*!

He smiled. I looked at the ground to avoid eye contact, as I sighed on the inside. My father's deficits never got easy to witness, no matter how many I had seen at that point. Then the nurse said, "And do you know your birth date?" Silence again. A moment of pause, and my mother filled in this lost information, and we continued on with the visit.

The neurologist met with us, and she asked my dad to clean his hands. She pushed the sanitizer towards him. "Here, Richard. Can you clean your hands?" she asked while looking directly at him.

I watched. I held my breath. I realized or assumed this was probably a test. A test of his mental acuity, as well as an ability to perform a simple, daily task. A test I'd seen him fail at home with me at the sink. How would he handle a pump bottle of sanitizer? He looked at her, at the bottle. She pushed it closer and coaxed him, "Richard, the hospital is full of germs today. Can you wash your hands?"

He took it with his right hand and awkwardly pushed down on the top with the same hand. The other hand did not meet to catch the sanitizer flowing out. The doctor helped him and moved his other hand under it. My dad just sat there with the sanitizer sitting in his palm, as if it was some mystery liquid, and he had to figure out what to do with it.

"Rub your hands together. Clean them," the doctor directed him patiently with a sense of calm.

Then, the most interesting thing happened. I was amazed. I was in awe. My father began to clean his hands the way you see a surgeon on TV clean his hands in a scrub room. He rubbed his hands while splaying his fingers open and scrubbing the insides. I had no idea what made him wash his hands the way he did that day. I didn't know if the doctor saying "hospital" triggered something or the words "germs," but something clicked, and he went back into that doctor mode for a few brief seconds in time. That was probably the only time I had and will ever witness him washing his hands as he had as a surgeon. My father washing his hands in a scrub room was something I had never witnessed, only something I secretly wished for at times. I would have loved to see my father do what he did best, operate on people, but that job doesn't lend itself to the watchful eyes of the public. Why couldn't they have operating theaters where people could come and watch a surgery happen like on TV? According to my dad, when I had asked a few years earlier, those didn't really exist anymore.

The neurologist just watched my dad, nodded her head, and made some notes. The visit continued, and finally, my mother told her she had plans to take my dad to the ocean soon for another visit, the same place we had gone the summer before. She said a caregiver would be accompanying them this time, along with their grandson, my son, Jacob. The neurologist smiled and said, "That's wonderful."

Then my mother asked, "What stage are we in here?" I felt bad that we discussed that in front of my dad. It was like saying, "Yup, you are on your way to the end. To die. All of your basic life skills will continue to deteriorate, and eventually you won't be able to use the bathroom, walk, cough, swallow, or breathe." The neurologist replied that it looked like the beginning of the "severe" stage. The final stage. Seeing my father struggle to remember his full name and use a bottle of sanitizer didn't make me question the doctor's judgment. My mother and I weren't that surprised to hear it, but it didn't make it any easier to hear it confirmed. My heart hurt hearing the confirmation. I took a sharp breath in, while I stood in the corner of the room close to the curtain, and I immediately wanted to wrap myself up in it and just cry. I felt bad for my mother, but I felt worse for my father and what he may still be able to understand at that point. For some reason, his career as a doctor always had me thinking he understood everything that was said in front of him. Yet, his expression and reaction to hearing that news was a blank stare straight ahead.

I began to really think hard about what that meant for my dad and how much time he had left. I had read online that the severe stage could last only one and half years before the patient died. It hadn't even been three years since my father's initial diagnosis, yet things were moving fast. Three years can feel like the blink of an eye or one hundred years at times. When I thought about how long my father had been living with Alzheimer's that was known, and possibly unknown to us prior to diagnosis, it truly was the "long goodbye" that I've heard other people comment about the disease.

The only other thing I remember from that visit was the doctor stating that my parents should do everything they want and make travel plans, as this would most likely be the last year my father would be able to do anything like that. After we left the exam room, my parents stopped at the family bathroom because my dad couldn't go unaccompanied anymore. He needed assistance with clothing, washing his hands, and directions. While they were in the bathroom, I just stood and watched all the people coming and going through the hospital halls. My father's appointment had me feeling numb at the gravity of the situation we were in, as well as where we were headed as he deteriorated. I smiled at people as they walked by and we made eye contact. My father's situation had made me feel even more sensitive to other people's life circumstances. I felt alone that day in my grief, standing in the hall but comforted by the idea that any one of those passersby could be facing the same or similar situation that was just unknown to me. Everyone had a battle they were fighting that day, seen or unseen.

18

few more months passed, and my father held steady in his disease. As the year came to a close, we would be faced with additional challenges beyond just my father's. The calendar was on the cusp of turning to 2020, and so we rang in the new year in style—with a hospital visit. My mother had taken a fall on Christmas Eve, and by New Year's Eve, her leg had progressed to a large, painful hematoma. The blood thinners she had been on for a few years had made her that much more delicate. By New Year's Eve, she needed to be seen, as things were looking and feeling worse for her. She secured a ride to the ER, and I stayed back at their home with my dad. Dad was scared, and I could tell he missed my mom the minute she left. He paced around looking out the window or pretended to search the kitchen for something to eat. He finally settled in a chair that faced the driveway, and he just sat and waited. I tried to tell him she wasn't returning the same way she left, that we were going to pick her up, but that didn't seem to affect his decision to stay seated. I tried to distract him and keep him occupied. "Want to watch a show?" I offered, trying to distract his mind from possibly focusing too much on worrying.

"Sure," he said, still staring out the window. At that point in his disease, my father had caregivers during the day a few times a week, for a few hours, but not that day, not on New Year's Eve. I was his caregiver in my mother's absence. I was a bit uneasy about it all. I was worried for my mom, and I was worried I wouldn't be able to keep my dad distracted enough. *What if he decided that was the day he was going to put up a fight about something?* He had never become combative, violent, or argumentative, but I knew it was a possibility with his disease.

After a few hours, my mom called to report things were going well, and she could go home soon. I told my dad, and he asked, "Is she okay?" I reminded myself I could still talk to him normally, so I attempted to explain without insulting him, all while trying to be cautious not to assume he understood everything or anything anymore.

I said she was going to get an X-ray. "Dad, you know

what an X-ray is, right?"

As usual, he sort of surprised me and said, "Yes, of course." *Phew.* For a moment I felt like it was Old Dad when he responded with a twinge of attitude that I might have insulted his intelligence. In the past, I would have felt offended by that, but that day I welcomed his tone, as it reminded me of the man he used to be, the doctor who wouldn't need to be reminded or questioned of his medical prowess.

When it was time to go get her, I said with elation and relief, "Mom can come home! Let's go get her!" He was delighted. He got up and quickly made his way to where I was. He stood at a dining room chair waiting for me to bring his coat and boots, like a little boy eager to go outside. I thought for a moment. I needed to remember where we were at with the disease. I needed to think for him and remind him of things that needed to be done before leaving the house. I said, "Dad, maybe you should use the restroom before we go. Come on. Let's go use the bathroom." He followed me, and I only had to help with his belt. *Phew.* Another hurdle I got past without my mom being around. I knew at times he needed more assistance in the bathroom, and as his daughter, I didn't feel totally comfortable in that role. I knew if push came to shove, and

I had to really help, I would, but if I could avoid it, I would. I felt bad feeling that way, but there had to be some limits still for my dad and I, if I could manage to maintain them. I got his coat and hat on him, and he pushed his own feet into his boots. We walked to the garage, and he climbed into the passenger seat and just sat. I buckled him into his seat. I apologized and then laughed and said with a sad attempt at a British accent, "Pardon me, sir," as I reached across his chest and lap to find the buckle. I never knew how he felt about the help that was given to him, but I always tried to respect him and not make a huge deal of it. I tried to lighten the mood. My constant goal was to never make him feel less than, stupid, or unaware. I did my best. I felt that if I made a little joke, it wouldn't seem so raw and so harshly apparent that I was helping him with a task that my children had mastered by the time they went off to kindergarten.

I think my mother welcomed the visit to the ER, as it was a break for her. She was taken care of, had no responsibilities except for herself, and her health was someone else's priority. As a mother, I understood this, and I tried to remain respectful of this for her. I still hurt for my parents that my dad, the doctor, couldn't accompany her to the ER and be her voice as he had been for so many years. A few months prior, my mother had gotten a cat bite and again, the blood thinners put her in a category that meant she needed to get to the ER immediately. That time, I took her while my dad stayed home. The ER doctor asked her who she lived with, and she said, "My husband. He has Alzheimer's, though, so my daughter came with me." She cried upon saying this. I choked back tears that day as well. I knew that was hard for her to say out loud, to admit, and most of all, to accept. That day in the ER exam room, while my mother said that through tears, I really felt as if life had shifted. My dad really wasn't there and wasn't able to be there to help, but I realized after that day, we got through it without him. My mother received the care she needed, and we did it together. It didn't change the fact she was missing my father at her side. She had lost her medical touchstone, her partner, but it proved she could do it on her own whether she wanted to or not. In some ways, I think it was harder to witness my mother not having my father with her because of his disease than if my father had actually died. My mother not only had the struggle of losing a man who still lived, but also the struggle of taking care of him while grieving him. I grieved for both of them, as I witnessed their relationship change and morph into something completely different than I had ever known. I witnessed my mother gain confidence in taking charge of her own health while my father slipped away into a battle with his, all while knowing that if he was healthy of mind, he would have been on the frontlines with my mother. I missed my father's medical expertise and confidence, but I also just missed him as my dad and my mom's partner. He wasn't gone, but he wasn't there. The level of pain and frustration that presented to me was unbearable at times, and I wanted to scream and cry, "It isn't fair! This is not how it was supposed to go!" I wished he was still Old Dad.

Reuniting my parents on New Year's Eve was bittersweet. I knew my father was relieved, but I think my mother just knew she was going back to her home and her responsibilities, with her own injury to slow her down. As we walked into the ER that night, there was a thin coating of snow in the parking lot. I held my dad's arm as we walked. If he fell and got hurt, I think my head would have exploded. Worrying about my mother and tending to my dad's current needs were all I could handle at that point. We walked through the automatic doors into the small, empty ER. In a small town, an ER looks more like a regular doctor's office. I had just been at an ER six days prior in my husband's small hometown with Hannah, as she had fallen on ice on Christmas Day and needed stitches in her chin. That year was ending with quite the bang. Within minutes, the nurse came out to get us, so we could meet my mother in her exam room. When we arrived, she was sitting and waiting for us. My dad's eyes lit up and, my mom's did too, but then her smile faded, as our arrival meant it was time to go home. Her leg hurt, but she did not have a suspected blood clot. However, she still needed a wheelchair to get out to the car. My anxiety grew, as now I was responsible for getting both of them out of the ER, into the car, and home. I looked around the room, trying to formulate a plan on how the rest of the night was going to go. It continued to snow outside. I fought back tears, as I looked at both of my parents who needed me. I could feel myself start to sweat with the stress of the situation that navigating the drive home in a snowstorm presented. I was a nervous driver for the most part, so the combination of factors that night made my anxiety level rise with each passing minute. I had two dependent adults to care for that night, and I hoped I wouldn't let either of them down. It was going to be slow and a team effort, but we made it. I had decided to leave my parents in the ER waiting room, together, while I went to get the car. I trusted my mother could manage my father mentally, and I knew my dad would not leave my mother's side. I also sort of winked and nodded at the secretary on the way out to the car, with a silent message of, "Keep an eye on them." My patience that I had attempted to master over the years as a mother came in handy. Gone were the days of sipping champagne, watching *Dick Clark*, and falling asleep on the couch early on New Year's Eve, for all three of us.

That night, it was a joint effort to put Dad to bed. We worked together to brush his teeth, wash his face, and change his clothes. My father could no longer remember what to do with a toothbrush, but he opened his mouth when I asked him to, and I maneuvered the toothbrush inside as best I could. I was used to brushing my kids' teeth when they were under the age of seven, but they were little bodies, and their heads were smaller and more moveable. I placed them in my lap like I was their dentist, or I could instruct them to say, "Ah," or, "Cheese," which meant close your teeth, but keep your mouth open. When I told my dad to say cheese, he said, "Cheese," and then closed his mouth. I probably let out a giggle through my exasperation with this, but I was used to people often not complying with me (as children often do). I needed to figure out different directions if this was going to be successful.

I sat at his feet and changed his socks, as my mother sat by and instructed. I said, "Dad, would you like some lotion?" I rubbed his feet, I looked up at him, and I felt as if I was giving back to him in the only way I could now. I helped keep his body clean, well-dressed, and groomed. I put his socks on him. No easy task on a grown man. He then thanked me. He always said thank you when anyone helped him do something he no longer could.

That night, I looked around and felt humbled for my parents, with my mother who was hurt and essentially incapacitated, and my father who was incapacitated in his own way. To see them like this was a wake-up call that life wasn't what it used to be. My parents were aging, and I was taking responsibility for them. I felt sorry for myself that I had to do this so soon in life, knowing that I had friends whose parents still took care of my friends and their children. I was in the reverse of that situation, and I felt as if my New Year's Eve party was going to be a pity party for one instead. I went from caring for my children to caring for my parents, within hours of each other. It was the same but different, all at once. I gave up celebrating New Year's Eve with Denis and my kids in order to care for my parents. I was resentful that I gave up family time, but also grateful I could, that my schedule and lifestyle allowed me to give time to my parents who needed me. So many conflicting emotions. I tucked in my dad, removed his glasses, and turned out the light. *Goodnight, Dad.* I eventually climbed into bed and checked my phone. My sisters sent texts that night, exclaiming, "Happy New Year!"

I finally wrote back, "Stop sending these!" I was mad. They realized the gravity of the situation and the state of emotional chaos I was in and finally texted back, "Sorry." I was jealous that they were probably cuddling with their significant others or partying with friends. They had helped Mom with Dad over Christmas while I celebrated with my husband's side in Vermont, so I tried to control my bitter feelings. They had been there when Mom fell and took care of her for the week following Christmas. I was still awake at midnight but not celebrating. I sat in bed listening for any noise from downstairs that indicated my parents might need me. I didn't sleep well that night, tossing and turning and holding my breath to see if I could hear any sounds. I welcomed the new year with sadness and anxiety, rather than the joy and hope for a fresh start.

The next morning, I got emotional while my parents ate breakfast that I had served them. I stood with my arms crossed and leaned up against the counter, while English muffins warmed to a crisp behind me. I paced around the kitchen, sighing audibly between spreading jelly on the muffins and pouring juice for my dad. My mom watched me from the table and could sense my tense attitude. "I feel like you don't want to be here," she said after a few minutes of my kitchen antics. I felt bad that she had sensed it, but I couldn't help it

I finally exploded. "I just can't sit here and watch you two be alone! This is so hard for me. You both need help right now, and I am terrified to leave you here when I go home later. I feel like you should move…" My mother had heard enough. She didn't want me to finish the sentence that would have ended with "…to a nursing home or assisted living." She asked me to stop and said their life was there, and no one was going anywhere.

I stepped away from the table and stared out the window. I struggled to fight the feeling inside to give them their independence, while knowing they needed me there then. I wanted to go home and see my kids and Denis. At that moment, caring for my parents eclipsed my usual exhaustion from my own children. I was emotionally and physically exhausted and had that kind of sleep hangover that comes with caring for a newborn or pulling an all-nighter in college, minus the alcohol. Loving someone so much you just want them cared for, but at the same time don't want to always have to be the one, but feel as if you should be the one to do it, was my inner struggle. I knew at that point that my parents needed more than just a caregiver a few hours a day. My parents needed overnight help. They needed someone to help my mom put my dad to bed and help get him up in the morning. I was worried, with my mother's leg and my father's dependency, that if they didn't have more help, that the situation would become even more dire. We managed to piece together the care for my parents between the daytime caregivers, my parents' cleaning woman who went above and beyond the call of duty, and me floating up through the weeks while my mother was healing. My mom and I sat one night in the living room while my dad slept, and she looked at me and said, "I know. I know we need more help; you are right. I'll have to figure it out. This isn't what I planned for our life. I hate having to see you stressed because of Dad and me. It's not fair." She said this while fighting back tears. I was relieved she was seeing my side in this situation. I knew I wasn't the only one suffering, and I knew none of this was easy for anyone, but it helped to hear my mother recognize the fact that she wasn't the only one affected by Dad's disease. My mother had it the hardest, and I knew that. I wanted to wipe it all away for her, but I couldn't. We had to face it. We had to grin and bear it, and it sucked.

As I lay in bed at night in the weeks following, I worried about my parents, and I could feel I was starting to crack. I could feel myself starting to slip into a hole of despair and loneliness. I felt alone in my journey with my parents. I had support from Denis and my sisters, but I needed more from someone else. Not Denis, not my friends, or my sisters. Denis was an amazing shoulder for me to lean on and always had a hug to offer, but I couldn't depend on him to give me the insight I was craving. I was looking for someone who was in the thick of it like me. I wanted to find another daughter whose father had Alzheimer's and was young and struggling like me to balance kids and parents and all the heartache. I wanted a person outside of my circle, someone who "got it." I had no friends who had parents with Alzheimer's. I had friends whose parents had cancer, diabetes, and other ailments, but not Alzheimer's. I needed to talk to someone my own age experiencing the same thing. I started to research support groups. I scoured the internet. I typed in things like "Alzheimer's support groups and caregiver support groups." Oh, that's right. I wasn't a caregiver... well, not one all the time. Oh, and I wasn't a spouse. And I wasn't the person suffering with Alzheimer's. My searches came up very thin in the area I lived in, and even so, the timing and locations were less than ideal for me. I was actually surprised at the lack of support for caregivers and family members in New Hampshire. I had to really dig to find anything, and I pride myself on my use of the internet. So how were others who were less savvy even finding any support?

I finally found a nursing home in the town over and visited their website, looking for any form of support. I called the number listed on their site, and an older woman with a kind and patient voice answered the phone. I explained my situation. She said, "Oh, we have a group that meets once a month on Wednesdays here at 2 P.M." *Wednesday. 2 P.M. Once a month.* I felt shut out. I have children. What if I also had a job? I started to realize these groups were for older people. Retired people. Caregivers who could bring their loved ones with them while they met with a group of their peers.

I said, "Well, I can see if I can make that work. I'm only forty. Will I feel silly that I'm coming on behalf of my dad who has early onset?"

She said, "No. Most are caregivers or spouses, but you will be fine." I hung up and cried a little. I cried out of relief. I was finally going to be able to share my story, breathe, and feel heard and understood. When I made that call, it was as if a weight had been lifted off my shoulders. I was relieved that I admitted I wanted to talk about this and get help from others. That act alone made me feel better. I had sought professional help in the past for anxiety and for struggling to process my miscarriages. This time, I wasn't ready to meet with a professional. I wanted to talk to other people who were going through what I was going through. I didn't want to just sit and vent to a therapist. I wanted to feel part of a group that understood and could empathize with me. I didn't want solutions or advice. I just wanted to feel less alone. I needed a support structure that consisted of people like me or at least felt like I did, watching their loved ones decline while standing by feeling helpless.

I never made it to the group meeting, as COVID soon crept into our world. It was as if a door was slammed shut in my face quickly, after someone had opened it and said, "Come on in!" I was frustrated and bummed that I wasn't able to do something that felt like a step in the right direction for my mental health. I struggled to accept it but was distracted by the chaos that COVID brought into our lives. My path to group healing had to be put on the back burner while other fires needed extinguishing instead, such as my children being home for the remainder of their school year.

I was proud of myself for making that step to find a place. It was time to think of myself. I wasn't giving up. I just had to find a new path for the time being. I turned to an old favorite of mine—yoga. I set up my little phone in my room, dimmed the lights, threw out my yoga mat, and stretched and breathed. I found a free yoga class on YouTube, and after dinner one night, I told Denis, "I am going upstairs, and I need thirty minutes to be alone." That translated to, "Do not let the kids bug me."

He nodded his head and said, "Yup! Got it." He knew I needed that time, and he was more than willing to make sure I was able to get it. He loved to tout the phrase, "Happy wife, happy life." I had to agree with him that the thirty minutes to myself attempted to fulfill that. A small thing, like yoga or a walk on the treadmill in the basement and a good cry, allowed me to get through a tough day or enough to release the stress I was feeling for the time being. Of course, coupled with texts to my sisters or friends, it worked. I felt more at ease, calmer, and able to handle my range of emotions. I realized I had the power to control my feelings, and working my mind and body made me feel that strength. I had to let out my tension in different ways, through tears, laughter, deep breathing, meditating, exercise, and of course, talking about what I was feeling. I still longed for that personal connection with a peer who was going through what I was at the time, but I had to realize that had to come later when the world was more able to provide that. I believed in things happening for a reason and that timing was everything. The new year had begun with a challenge, and I attempted to take it on the best way I could.

19

---◆—◆—◆---

Amonth later, and things were finally in a *good* place. A better place. A manageable place. My mother's leg was improving, and my dad still had his caregivers for a few hours a day, the perfect respite for my mother. My father's current caregivers were excellent. One in particular was extremely motivated, patient, kind, and caring. She walked outside with my dad every time she worked with him, and her attentiveness was admirable. She read to him, watched TV with him, helped in the bathroom, and dressed him. She made sure he drank enough water and sometimes even brought an activity for them to do together. She was like the Mary Poppins of adult caregivers.

I was able to carve out time to visit, and we could breathe a bit since the caregiver was around helping with Dad and easing some stress for my mother. Often Henry accompanied me while Hannah and Jacob attended school. One day, the news reported there was a respiratory virus running rampant in China. *This will never get past our borders,* I remember thinking. The news was more cautious. It seemed more real. The warnings started coming more often, and people began dying on the West Coast in the United States. I called my mom one day and said, "Mom, you should be careful." My mother's auto immune disease didn't take kindly to viruses, and this one sounded troubling. All I could imagine was something happening to my mother and me having to care for my father in her absence. I was terrified. I knew their plan was for him to stay at home. Forever. There was no option to move him out to a nursing home. My mother had already shot down my idea for assisted living. My instinct was right, as the virus kept making its way across the country like a wave that keeps moving in with the tide. Life got a little more difficult. My children began attending school online from our dining room, and Henry, being four at the time, needed more attention to be kept entertained while Hannah and Jacob attempted to focus during classes. Not only did I have them to keep focused, but visiting my parents at this point was actually dangerous. We could bring an illness to them that could actually kill them. I felt as though my hands were tied. I definitely felt as if I had to choose between them, but the virus made that choice for me by limiting my interaction. Sometimes the pull to see my parents, yet stay home to care for my children, felt so intense I wanted to scream. And sometimes I did. I lost my patience. I lost my cool. I cried and shouted at Denis who continued to work in his office a few towns away. "How can you just keep going there every day while the world shuts down around us?" I said between sobs. I just wanted him to stay home and work as it seemed everyone else was doing. It didn't feel safe or right for him to keep leaving and returning daily. He assured me of the precautions being taken at his work and his concern for all of us. The virus was still in a very new stage in our country, and the unknowns made me insane. I lived in my house in a bubble with my children, avoiding the outside world for weeks. I knew some of that was my anxiety creeping in, but also, I was always thinking about my parents. I felt as if Denis working in his office put me at an unfair risk that, in turn, limited my access to my parents. I hated having to feel as if I couldn't do both—be with my kids and my parents. I wanted to be able to swoop in and help my parents when a caregiver didn't show up for their shift, but the pandemic made me feel like an outsider looking in. And sometimes,

I was literally outside, looking in at them. I was trapped behind glass waving because I wasn't sure if I harbored a silent virus.

We tried to FaceTime, but my father was confused most of the time. Watching his face try to understand where we were was depressing. He looked around or stared at my face on the screen, questioning, I am sure, the reality of it all. My sisters and I even tried FaceTiming as a family. I don't think that was a good idea either, as our voices actually all sound the same. It must have been some sort of crazy echo to my dad, as we all tried to talk over each other. Why did life have to get more complicated? More confusing? Anything out of the ordinary for my father just didn't seem fair.

Two months into the pandemic, I finally decided to visit my parents. I felt awful they would be alone for Easter. I told my mom I was going to make ham and deliver it. Window visits were becoming popular for seeing those outside your household, so we planned one for Easter. It was a gloomy April day. A blanket of gray clouds covered the sky, and the wind was particularly vicious that day. We wore jackets over our Sunday best. I am not sure why I told my children to dress up that day, since church was not holding mass, and we were only seeing my parents from the outside. It just felt like a tradition that we should try and keep since nothing else felt normal anymore. My dad sat in a rocking chair with a blanket on his lap, and he was positioned right in front of the glass door to the outside. He looked more decrepit. Confused. Again, I felt discouraged we had to even do that, as I wondered what he thought of it all. I would never know what was actually going through his mind. We talked through the glass. I tried to shout, so he could hear me. I turned to Denis a few times and quietly commented on how messed up this whole thing was becoming. Finally, my mother opened a window, and she leaned out while talking to us, while my dad sat behind the glass door just staring. I was more than frustrated. It was bad enough to wonder whether he remembered or knew me, but I was talking to him from outside with my family. With his grandchildren. The grandchildren who should be seated around the dining room table with their grandparents while we all enjoyed an Easter meal. My children wanted to go inside. It was cold. They "had to pee," of course. I instructed my mother to open the walk-out basement door, so we could use the basement toilet. My kids ran around the back of the house and came back after a few minutes.

This isn't fair! I just kept thinking. Dad must think he's hallucinating. *God, I wish he wasn't sick.* I was dying to know what he thought of all of this. I wanted his opinion, his guidance, and his reassurance. We were floating in a sea of fear, and our captain had abandoned ship. His career as a doctor was the only solace for me at times when I tried to explain our distance during a visit. "Dad, there is a *pandemic.*" I waited to see if the word "pandemic" rang a bell, lit up his eyes. Did it register? "This is ridiculous. I know," I sometimes commented to him.

Finally, toward the end of the month, I realized if caregivers and the cleaning woman could enter my parents' home, then so could I. My kids had been home for weeks at that point, and Denis was being as safe as he could at work. I told my mother I would wear a mask, though. Masks were becoming a norm, and in some cases, a requirement, in stores, offices and other places of business. I showed up, cleaned my hands, and entered my parents' house. I even put socks on when I got to their house, so my bare feet didn't bring any germs from my own house. It had been over two months since I had been inside their home. My dad sat at the dining room table. I walked in. His eyes lit up. "Hi, Dad! I am here!" I said, smiling behind my mask. He got up and walked to me and stood close.

He said, "What have you been doing?" Did he

question my mask? Did he think I was someone else? Did he think he was back in the operating room?

I said "I know this is silly, but I need to wear it, so you and Mom don't get sick." He didn't respond. He didn't ask any questions. I didn't want him to think *he* was sick, but rather that I was protecting him. A silver lining, one silver lining, was that while we all had to wear masks around a potentially confused dementia patient, my father was most likely a pro at seeing people with masks and learning to communicate behind them. Maybe being a surgeon made all of this not so strange. Maybe he felt as though this was what he was used to, not from his daughter, but if anyone can understand someone behind a mask, it's the man who spent his career behind one. He spent countless hours standing over a patient while wearing a mask, teaching his students and working with colleagues, all while his and their mouths and noses were covered. His ears were attuned to listen, rather than read lips. His eyes spoke volumes, and I believe he looked at others' eyes to see their reaction as well. It was the one comfort I held onto that maybe, just maybe, these masks were not a total kick in the gut as they seemed to be for everyone else. The man who was historically behind the mask tending to a patient was now the patient. And I, ironically, looked like the doctor.

We sat down, and I pulled my mask down briefly and said, "See? It's me, Drea." He smiled back at me. I never knew what he really thought of my mask. He just smiled when I made a joke about it or referenced it. I kept my visit brief, and I touched his shoulder when I left. I didn't hug him or my mother. It was torture for me not to hug my parent's goodbye. It was like we were acquaintances not family, disconnected, unloving. It didn't feel like me. It didn't feel like *us*. I had to remember that I was doing that to protect them and keep them safe. The visit alone was risky enough, but I had to weigh the importance of visiting my dad versus staying away, and visiting won for me. I knew my time with my dad was limited in general, and my mother and I decided the risk was worth it.

When visitors were not allowed at nursing homes in the area due to the pandemic, I was grateful my father was still at home. I was able to visit whenever I wanted without restrictions or rules, other than the ones my mother and I decided were appropriate. Another silver lining.

20

I continued to visit and help my parents in 2020, but a visit to my parents provided as much solace as it did pain for me. I enjoyed seeing them and checking in on them, regardless of what I did while I was there. I loved my parents, but every time I saw my dad, I struggled to put myself back together. When I would arrive home, I would emotionally collapse. My head and heart would need a day or two to recoup. I found that fresh air, exercise, and, surprisingly, my children would be what pulled me out of any funk I may have felt after a visit. Some days, I stuck my headphones in my ears, grabbed the dog and her leash, and told Denis or Jacob I was going for a walk. The music and the movement made me feel alive and able to process how I was feeling. My children would run to me when I got home from my walk as if I had been gone for years, rather than twenty minutes. Their innocence and oblivious nature, especially Henry's, to what was really happening was a welcome relief. Jacob, being twelve at the time, observed my mood or knew where I had been and asked the most questions. He wanted to know how Papa and GG were doing. He knew my dad had Alzheimer's and had seen firsthand the devastation it was causing for my father.

Jacob was the one who remembered my dad before he became the different version of himself. He was my father's first grandchild. My father's first "boy." Jacob and my dad shared a connection and love for tractors. The year Jacob was in fourth grade, he had a teacher whose mother had Alzheimer's. Often, she explained to the students what this meant. She might share a story about how her mother asked, over and over again, for some tea. Jacob knew it meant that as people aged, they forgot, so when my father was diagnosed with Alzheimer's, I told him, eventually. I tried to explain to him and Hannah that, "Papa has something wrong with his brain." Ultimately, I knew Hannah was too young to understand at the age of four, and Jacob was somewhat aware, but for him, his grandfather didn't have noticeable differences yet. I did tell them once that if they saw me sad or upset, it was probably about Papa and that I would be okay. I didn't want them to worry or always think it was something they had done or not done. I tried to emotionally prepare them for my own possible breakdowns. Telling people my father had Alzheimer's was difficult because every time I said it out loud, it made it more real. It would take a while, a few years, for me to be able to say it without my voice cracking. I was so grateful Jacob had that teacher that year because when I told him, he said, "Oh yeah. I know what that is." Jacob was only nine when my father was diagnosed, but he was already so wise. He had more grace and compassion with my father than some adults. He was patient and sweet, and his experience as a big brother to Hannah and Henry seemed to shine when my dad needed the same guidance. Jacob often offered to "watch Papa" while someone else left the room or went to make a meal. He wasn't afraid or intimidated. My dad had played the typical grandfather role with Jacob in the early years of Jacob's life, before my dad's disease showed its truth. Jacob loved him for who he had been and who he was now. He held no judgment. Just pure love. He traveled with my parents on their last trip to the ocean the summer after we had gone as a family. My mother had just wanted to take him, my father, and a caregiver. My dad had wandered to Jacob's room in the middle of the night, obviously confused. Jacob didn't miss a beat and walked him back to his room. He knew my dad needed his guidance, understanding, and patience. Many adults who met Jacob during that time commented on how wise and wonderful he was with my dad. I was proud to see that their relationship carried on through the decline. I was amazed that Jacob, being so young, had an innate ability to be so gentle and caring with my father, considering Jacob had no experience around someone with this disease. Seeing Jacob like this, with my father, gave me so much hope for Jacob to grow into a caring and compassionate adult and maybe father himself one day. I often smiled to myself, knowing he was my son and that he was becoming a wonderful little human. Those were the times that all my commitment, energy, time, and love to my children as a stay-at-home mom felt worthwhile, and maybe, just maybe, I had something to do with how he was turning out. Children can teach us a lot about love. About what *really* matters. He was sad when I updated him on my father's decline, and he often hugged me if he saw I needed one. As sad as it was, my father's illness allowed Jacob to see and understand the world through a lens of compassion and maturity, and for that I was grateful.

Hannah was the one who didn't remember my father before his illness and was only four when he was diagnosed. She knew my father as a quiet man. Their interactions were mostly smiles and the occasional question from him earlier in his disease like, "How's school?" or, "What have you been up to?" One day when Hannah was seven, we were visiting my parents together. She came next to me, and I said to my dad, "Do we look alike?" Hannah and I both had the same color of brown eyes and a very similar shade to our brown hair. He just stared at me. Then at her. *Okay, I'll try this again.* "Does she look like me when I was little?" Nothing. No response. He kept staring. Finally, I said, "Isn't she pretty?"

He finally replied, "Beautiful." Hannah and I both turned to each other and smiled.

Out of my three children, I felt the saddest for Hannah. She never knew my dad like Jacob, and their bond wasn't as strong because my father declined just as Hannah was becoming conscious of her own life. Hannah reminded me of myself, trying to get to know a man who was at arm's length. I suppose the difference was she was accepting of this and didn't know what she was missing, Old Papa. She simply loved him for what she knew, not what she remembered or hoped for the future. Hannah was the type of child who waited to be engaged in a conversation, so the silence between her and my father was mutual. Their minds were built similarly in Hannah's enjoyment for math and love of reading. She had a competitive spirit and a love of sports, so her mind and body were always active and churning out new ideas. She was content in the silence between them and sometimes just sat there, studying my father's face. She didn't seem uncomfortable or worried, just present in the moment. She was always the quiet, thoughtful one. She recorded herself playing "Happy Birthday" on the piano or created an elaborate drawing and wrote, "To: Papa. From: Hannah," on it and shyly brought it along with her on a visit. Hannah inspired me to accept "what is" rather than "what was" or "what could have been" and embrace it.

Henry was the one who surprised me the most. He was an infant when my father was diagnosed and grew up around him more than the others had, since my parents didn't move to New Hampshire until Jacob was six and Hannah was two. Henry brought innocent joy with him whenever he was around. He loved going to visit my parents, and there were many times I questioned if he was actually the only one my dad did remember. Henry would enter the room and my dad's eyes would light up. Henry might even get a laugh out of him. When Henry was two, and my father was still walking, he used to walk us to the door before we left. Henry hugged my mom goodbye and ran back to me. I said, "Henry, go give Papa a hug, too!" Henry hesitated then started toward my dad. My father knelt down, put his arms out, and picked Henry up. My eyes widened. My father hadn't been initiating hugs for some time now, but for some reason, Henry brought out something in him. Watching him interact with my children made me so happy, even if it was for a brief moment. That moment of being a grandfather. I looked at my mother, and we both just gave that look to each other that said, "Aw." It was a moment when things felt completely as they should, but it was fleeting, and I knew that. I enjoyed the interaction, my shoulders relaxed, and my heart felt full. I doubt Henry or my dad will ever remember it, but I will.

Henry and my father had a lot in common. At times, they had similar challenges. Neither of them could tie shoes, put on a jacket, or make their own meals. Henry mastered a skill, and I'd call my mother to rejoice. She celebrated with me and then usually followed it with a similar defeat for my father. We were both giving care and facing similar obstacles. Henry talked in longer sentences, while my father shortened his. Henry finally dressed himself but wore his pants backward. My mother said the same about my father. We laughed, but it wasn't truly funny when the laughter faded. We knew the truth in those laughs were just us trying not to feel the sting of reality in those moments.

While Jacob and Hannah challenged me, and I fought not to worry about my parents, Henry would do something only a toddler can do. He provided an innocence and easy-going nature that only required a snack or a diaper change. I could hold Henry tight and snuggle him and bury my head in his warm, soft skin and just know I was holding onto life. A life that was continuing to develop, grow, learn, and advance with age. Henry aged forward, as my father aged backward.

Henry could lighten a mood. Henry was my comic relief most of the time. If we were all sitting around watching my dad struggle to feed himself or falling asleep at the table, Henry would pipe in with some funny saying or comment.

"I'll have a mustard sandwich, Mom!" Henry exclaimed with his hands folded while seated at the table one day.

"What? Just mustard?" I asked with a shock to my voice.

He responded completely seriously, "Yes!" My mother laughed, I laughed, and the world was okay in that moment; the world went on. Once, Henry was upstairs at my parents' house and found an old Elmo doll that had belonged to one of my sisters. Elmo made his way down the stairs way before Henry did, and Henry shouted, "Look out below!" My father was at the table, saw Elmo arrive, and started to chuckle. A smile was great. A laugh was a miracle, at that point, for my father. Henry often dressed in costumes at home or watched fairytales. He always wanted to be the character in the movie, and one day it was the movie *Tangled*, and he wanted to be Rapunzel. He didn't have long hair, but he managed to figure out a way. He brought me a long piece of toilet paper and a hair tie, stood in front of me, and said, "Mom, put this in my hair so I can look like Rapunzel." So I did. I just accepted him for who he was and what made him happy. I laughed as he ran out of the room with the toilet paper trailing behind him.

He always brought a light of hope in all of this. His birth marked the start of the clock for my father's decline when I tried to remember how long my dad had been sick. I could calculate it quickly by doing the math with the year Henry was born. I began to realize how lucky I was that I had a positive event in the same year that there was such a negative one. It was a balance. Henry's life carrying on helped to remind me that life goes on and to focus on what was ahead, not always what was gone.

21

One day, while we remained hunkered down in our home during the pandemic, Jacob found old home videos on minidiscs from a few years prior. We put them in the DVD player and started to watch. It was a Christmas video from about six years before my dad's diagnosis. Jacob was only two years old, and my dad was showing him the train he had set up under the tree. My father lay on the ground with Jacob, watching the train go around and around the track. Then I heard it— my father's full belly laugh. I told Amy a few weeks later I had found the DVD and heard Dad laugh, and she said, "You mean his hyena laugh?"

"Oh, my God, yes. That's exactly what he sounds like," I responded, laughing myself. She was right. When my dad laughed, when he thought something was truly funny, he would laugh and it would build up, sounding like a hyena.

I took a deep breath when I heard his laugh on the video. It had been a few years since I had heard this signature laugh of my father's. I teared up. How different life was then. How quickly things had changed. It had been almost four years since his diagnosis, yet at times, it felt as if only four days had passed. Time was moving quickly. Like Denis said to me one day, while I stood in the kitchen crying over how fast things were progressing with my dad, "Drea, the days are long, but the years are short. It's like us raising the kids. When we look back, we can't believe how fast time has flown sometimes." Denis was right. Some days felt so long in the parenting world, and some days felt so long in the world of watching my father decline.

While our loved ones' memories are stolen from them, so are our memories of our loved ones, the way they *were*. In the face of Alzheimer's, a new person often emerges, a different personality or attitude in the patient. We long for the old days, for the person we once knew. Our memories begin to blur between the "old" person and the "new" person. I had a difficult time trying to remember my dad before his diagnosis because my dad had changed. His physical demeanor and looks had changed, some with age, some with the disease. His walk was now a shuffle, and his eyes were often softer and less focused. He acted differently. He was more mellow and very quiet, but he was always polite and grateful and concerned for others. He could not carry a conversation of more than a few words and often those words were only "yes" or "no." I had forgotten the sound of his voice. One day, Henry asked me, "Why did Papa lose his voice?" I was shocked by his question. Henry, being the tender age of four, *had noticed*.

I simply responded, "Papa has a disease." It was enough for Henry, and it was all I could manage to explain. I had a voicemail from my dad from about four months prior to his dementia diagnosis and had saved it. It was a message just calling to see how I was. He said my name, said I could call him if I wanted, and at the end, said he hoped I was having a great day. I kept it and listened to it whenever I felt down or just felt like hearing him talk to me, especially as time went on, and he lost his gift of words. When he progressed and only spoke once in a while and attempted to speak, I shushed those around me. I needed to hear whatever he was going to say. Did I expect it to be profound or earth shattering? No. I just wanted to hear my father say something, anything. Any way to get inside his head and his heart. He told stories sometimes about his past, and I often already knew them, but as time ticked on, the stories weren't as discernible and often sounded like, "That guy did things," or, "When I did that thing where people went." If my mother or sisters were around, we tried our best to remember his life and match what he was saying to the right story, the right memory. My dad was on a train of thought, and I had to stay on board, or I was never going to get where he was trying to take me.

During a visit one day, my dad and I chatted, and the caregiver sat and listened. I commented, "Isn't the view beautiful?" as I looked out at the mountains in the distance and the hill as it descended downward.

My father responded, "She found it," and pointed to me. I knew what he was trying to say, so I further clarified.

"I think he means I found the property. The land." I went on to explain that years before my parents built this house, they had purchased the land based on a phone call and a drive by, from me checking out the listing. It was six acres on an old ski hill that was for sale, and Denis and I had visited the property. Once we parked and I had gotten out to see the view, I called my parents right away and said, "This is the one. You are going to love it." They trusted me enough and, days later, bought the land that would eventually be the spot for their retirement. My father repeated the line about me "finding it," a few times when

I met a new caregiver. If he attempted to tell that story to a new caregiver with me there, I took it as a sign that he knew who I was that day.

He said "thank you" when I visited or if I helped him do something. He said "I'm sorry," even when he didn't need to apologize, but felt he had inconvenienced someone in some way. One day, when I visited, and a caregiver was there, he went into the basement to find my mom. He followed his caregiver back up the stairs, and she got to the top, turned to me, and said, "I just love your dad. He's so sweet. I just tripped up the stairs, and he asked me if I was okay." My heart melted hearing that. So many caregivers I met or spent time with gushed over how wonderful my dad was to them or how easy he was to care for. Observing my father with other people in this way was enriching and helped me realize maybe this "new man," who was seemingly helpless and lacked words, was actually someone still to be admired and imitated in the way he gently lived his life. He was always polite and well-mannered as Old Dad, but wasn't as observant as others, as I am sure he was preoccupied with his career or whatever else was zooming through his constantly busy mind. New Dad still seemed to honor his doctor's oath of "do no harm," in probably the only way he could, by still looking out for people's well-being. Often, he listened to a conversation between my sisters and me, or my mother and me, and he commented, "Are you okay?" with a genuine concern to his voice. I always assured him that I was, and that we were all okay.

My mother shared with me moments that caught her off guard. One night on a phone call, she told me, "Your dad said I was a 'good cook' tonight and patted my hand." My mother beamed through the phone at this, and I could hear the lightness in her voice. Like me, she cherished any moment that my dad's lucidity returned or if he made a comment that was direct and thoughtful, just for her. It was her reminder that my dad was still there, that he still knew her, or at least appreciated the things she did for him, such as cook a delicious meal.

A popular activity of ours when I visited was to go out for a walk. Depending on the weather and season, I helped him dress appropriately. If it was winter, he wore a Scottish cap, a scarf, gloves, and a heavy hunter green jacket that had zippers and snaps. At first, he fiddled with the snaps, usually snapping them out of order. I reached, grabbed his hands, and lowered them, gently saying, "That's okay, Dad. Let's get this zipped up first so you don't freeze out there." He usually gave in and let me take over. I placed his gloves on him, and this was my favorite part. It was my test to see how much of Old Dad was going to shine through. *How many times as a surgeon did he put gloves on?* For months into his disease, he easily found the finger holes, slipped his hands in, and pulled them tight. I imagined this is how he did it back then, preparing for surgery, and I was comforted. Eventually, there was a day he needed help to find the right spot for all his fingers. It was like when I dressed my kids in gloves for the first time, trying to guide them and getting frustrated when their thumbs tried to cram in with their forefingers. I turned to my mother after a few minutes and said, "Maybe Dad could try mittens?" My mother was already aware and had anticipated this might happen.

"Yup. I already got him some. They are in the closet." My mother was always one step ahead for my dad as his caregiver.

When I put them on his hands, I made sure not to make it about him not being able to put his gloves on, but instead I said, "These are going to be so much warmer for your hands." And off we went. The wind made my dad's nose run, and sometimes he laughed at that. The last time we walked together, my father seemed unsure of himself. I offered my arm, and he accepted it that time. Unlike other times, we didn't carry a conversation. I made a few comments on the houses we passed or the weather, but for the most part, my dad kept his eyes ahead, and he walked as if it was a task he had to focus to complete. We no longer stopped and enjoyed the view. He wanted to get back inside. Instead of getting upset, I accepted that this was what he could tolerate, and it was better than nothing.

Those were the moments I realized my father was still teaching me. New Dad and Old Dad didn't have to be totally separate men in my mind. Maybe he had changed physically, mentally, and emotionally in some ways, but he still guided me. He was teaching me patience, humility, and compassion. His mission to educate was still being fulfilled, even as a patient. It wasn't necessarily information you learned from a textbook or a class lecture, but they were lessons that one can only learn through experience. When he stood before my mother in the entrance to the bathroom one day and could barely stand to get out of his wheelchair, and I held him to try and coax him in there, he taught me compassion. The compassion to care for someone else who could no longer care for themselves in the most humbling of ways. I was used to helping my children with their basic needs and caring for them when they were sick, but as I cared for my father, an adult, I felt myself changing. I was no longer just a mother of young children. I was a daughter of a dependent, vulnerable adult, and I felt I could see a different side to life. It opened my eyes wider to the world beyond just parenthood. He taught me that love goes beyond hugs, or gifts, or saying, "I love you." He taught me love is shown in the way you help others and treat others with gentleness and consideration beyond your own needs. I started to feel that I was at a lucky age of physical and mental independence. I wasn't a child who needed caring for, yet I wasn't an elderly adult who needed caring for either. I felt strong and able-bodied and with that, a sense of duty to my fellow humans to look out for them while I could.

Those experiences taught me to become a more concerned and empathetic person when I saw a stranger struggling or an older person looking confused in a parking lot, as it happened at Target one day. A woman walked slowly, looking for her car, and turned to me and said, "I could have sworn I parked it right here." Instead of laughing it off as I might have in the past, I offered to help her look for it. I stopped, and I took the time to help and understand. I remembered that people may appear healthy or okay but could be battling something that wasn't easily apparent, like my father was. I began to try to let judgment slip away a bit. I began to give people the benefit of the doubt. If someone followed too closely on the road, maybe they were trying to get to an ailing parent or racing home to their children, as so often the case seemed to be for me now. That person looking confused in a parking lot could have been my dad, and someday, that person could be me. My father was still a father to me. He was guiding me on a journey of love, acceptance, and selflessness. To love him for who he was and who he had become. As a parent, you love your children unconditionally, and I was learning to love my father without conditions or expectations. I was letting go of what I wanted and learning to love and embrace what I had in New Dad.

22

When Jacob was two years old, he walked in my room one day and said, "Mommy, I just ate my medicine!" The smell of grape-flavored children's Tylenol wafted toward me. "Oh, my God!" I shouted. I ran downstairs to find an empty bottle lying on his little craft table. I hadn't realized he had grown tall enough to reach his medicine off the counter. I immediately called poison control to be reassured the amount he had eaten was safe, based on his age and weight. My next call was to my mother, who then had my father call me from his office. I needed his reassurance, his voice to tell me what to do. To my surprise, he just laughed when I told him of the day's traumatic event.

"Dad! Why are you laughing? Is Jacob going to have permanent liver damage? What should I look for? Worry about?" I frantically rattled off my questions of concern.

"Nothing. He will be fine. He might take a nap for you. That's about it," my father said with a laugh that faded into his serious voice, as he realized I was genuinely afraid. He used his humor to diffuse the situation. I must have inherited that from him. There was nothing to worry about. I just needed to hear him tell me that.

***

The calls and texts from my mother started coming faster and more frequently, as winter relented to spring, but the pandemic still held us in its grip. Most mornings, my mother texted my sisters and me a greeting, or a "good morning." It was her way to let us know she and Dad had survived the night and were functioning in the morning. Survived may be a dramatic word, but many times it was the word I used because I just wanted to know they were alive. I needed to know the night hadn't brought a fall or another event that would render my mother incapable and my father helpless in its occurrence. I went to bed every night and said a prayer that they would be okay. It began to really scare me that they lived alone. There came a time when I would receive a text or call saying Dad wouldn't get out of bed. One morning, my mother called, hysterical. "Can you tell Dad he needs to sit down in the wheelchair?

Just tell him," she said with a breathlessness and panic. Then she put the phone to his ear.

"Mom? What? What do I say? Dad? Can you sit down? Dad? Please sit in your chair for Mom," I said with a lack of confidence as the words came out. I wasn't sure that what I was saying was what she needed or he needed. I felt ridiculous saying it.

My mother got back on the line. "Okay. That worked, thank you," she said, her voice calmer, more relieved.

I guess my dad needed to hear it from someone else sometimes. She said my sister, Liza, and I had voices he responded to more than my mom's. Amy lived in a time zone that was an hour earlier; otherwise, I think she would have gotten the same call. Some days, I would be sitting on my screened-in porch, drinking my morning coffee, convincing my father to sit in his wheelchair, while my children ran around screaming and yelling in the background. It was sometimes a chaotic scene both on *and* off the phone. I wanted to hear what my mother was saying and concentrate, but my children made it increasingly difficult. I would close the slider doors to my porch and pray they wouldn't come barreling through them for the next few minutes. They often found me and pulled open the door, acting as if I had purposely hid from them.

"Mom! I need you! I need a drink! Why did you shut this?" one of them would ask while looking at me with a look of pure surprise.

I whispered, "I'm on the phone!"

"With who?" they whispered back. It didn't matter. They needed a drink, a channel changed, a snack, or to recruit me to referee their recent fight with a sibling. I felt bad for my mother that we were being interrupted, and I felt bad for myself that I couldn't have five minutes alone, even if it was to tell my dad to stand up or sit down. My patience wore thin, I felt my heart pound, and I eventually shouted, "Will you just leave me alone for a few minutes?!?" while my children took the hint and slinked away, heads down, as they slowly closed the slider. I felt like a bad mother and an inattentive daughter in those moments.

My father was getting harder and harder to move, and my mother was getting exhausted from the physical labor he demanded of her. She was doing almost everything for him at that point, and evenings and mornings were the hardest. She was on her own during those times, and there was no assistance or respite. The caregivers didn't arrive until 10 A.M. at the earliest. My mother was tired, physically and mentally. My father needed assistance with everything. She brushed his teeth, washed his face, changed his clothes, and physically put him into bed. He had forgotten how to lie down or, at least, what he was supposed to do when he got into bed. My mother told me sometimes my father would lay diagonally in the bed, and when she would go to bed a few hours after him, she would have to literally move him so she had room to crawl into bed. She had to push or pull him to one side. After a few minutes of that, I am sure it drained my mother completely. My mother called me one evening and said, "It just took me an hour to convince your father to lie down in bed." My heart hurt for my mother. I knew what it was like to put a small child to bed, and by the day's end, I was wiped. I wanted my children to go to bed immediately without a fight, without having to convince them. I can only imagine my mother felt the same, with an added thirty years, and the strength and size of an adult to handle. I was exhausted just listening to her describe her frustration. I knew she was tired physically and mentally, and she was tired of repeating herself, instructing my father to do things and making all the decisions for everything. Her strength, both emotionally and physically, astounded me at those times. Not once did she mention giving up on my father. She expressed her desire for a break, for a night away, but quickly tucked that thought to bed and persevered. I would say, "Let's go back to the ocean, just me and you some day. We can leave everyone behind!"

She would laugh and say, "Yeah… someday."

One of the phone calls was in the middle of a sunny, warm May day. The grass was green, and the air was breezy. The pandemic didn't change the seasons or keep the sun from shining. The kids were running in and out of the house between bike riding and playing soccer in the yard. She called and said, "Do you have a few minutes? I need to talk to you about something serious." If my mother said this, I knew she meant she needed some undivided attention from me. She told me Dad wouldn't get out of bed that morning and he seemed different, weaker. She had called his doctor, and they discussed hospice. *Hospice.* To me, hospice meant he was going to die soon. My only knowledge of hospice was that it was a place you went or a service that came to you within the last few days or maybe weeks of life to help you die peacefully.

"What? Really? Why?" I rapidly fired the questions, one after another. My heart began to pound, and my head felt as if it was spinning. I had to take a deep breath after I realized I had been holding it. I couldn't believe how quickly my father seemed to be declining. I panicked a bit, feeling as if I wanted more time with him. That I needed to be with him more. Hospice felt like the end, and I wasn't ready to give in to the feeling of relief that hospice brought so many people after a long struggle or battle. I didn't deny to myself that my father was going to die. I knew that Alzheimer's was terminal, but I didn't feel ready to accept it so soon.

My mom explained that the doctor suggested it based on the level of assistance my father needed and then asked me what I thought.

"What do I think? I don't even know." I knew my dad struggled to do most things, all things, alone. He could feed himself, sometimes, though often awkwardly. At times, he would forget to use a utensil or would ask how to eat a sandwich. He would just sit there staring at his plate, until someone reminded him what to do or handed him his food. He had been progressing quickly over the last few months especially. I didn't know if it was the lack of visitors due to the pandemic or just the coincidental timing of his disease and its natural progression that made his decline seem more pronounced. "Mom, if hospice means you get more assistance with Dad, then do it." The notion of putting Dad in a nursing home or both of my parents in an assisted living facility together had been discussed already. I had gently suggested it more than once but knew it would never happen. This was another moment I wanted to address it but knew it would not be received well. My mother was committed to keeping my father at home. She had spent endless amounts of money on supplies, caregivers, and most of all, she repeated over and over again, "I promised your dad I would never do that. I can't leave him." She found a way to do it on her own, even if it meant turning their house into a small, private, one-patient hospital. She knew caring for my dad was only getting more strenuous, time consuming, and often times, extremely humbling in the care he now required that, many times, only a loving spouse could take on, as no one else may feel comfortable who wasn't properly trained. I told my mom I thought hospice sounded like the next best step. She said, "Okay," with a sigh of relief, yet a hint of defeat. Her voice was calm and quiet, but also melancholy. There's no shame in asking for help. Hospice was extra, doctor-approved help, but it also sounded like the end of the road to my mother. They would be able to get overnight care as well. She wasn't ready to lose my dad. At times, I often thought, *She will never be ready.* How can anyone ever actually be ready to lose their loved one? You can prepare, but ultimately, none of us truly know how we will react to another person dying, until it actually happens. I looked up hospice after our conversation, and it was very common for Alzheimer's patients to enter hospice and stay with hospice for months, even years. The level of care needed, and the fact that Alzheimer's is a terminal illness, will qualify a patient, regardless of the time a doctor believes they have left. That made me feel a little better to know my father didn't have a set time left on Earth. The time left would be met with palliative care, and this would ensure quality of life, not necessarily quantity.

The sunny day and the idea of hospice presented conflicting feelings of peace and relief, coupled with a depressing guilt for me. Just a few nights before, I had sat on the same porch on a warm evening, keeping my hands busy by crocheting a blanket for a pregnant neighbor. I crocheted at times to ease my own anxiety, something I had started when I got pregnant with my daughter and worried every day her pregnancy would end in a third miscarriage. Denis sat across from me in another chair on his computer, and the kids were sleeping. His phone dinged from an incoming text. "Who is that?" I asked, being nosey.

"It's time! You have to go! Shannon's in labor!" Denis exclaimed, as if he was a proud uncle or grandfather.

"What? Oh my God! Eek! Okay! Um… I am not done with my blanket!" I said, as I threw it on the chair and stood up with my eyes wide. I laughed like it actually mattered whether the blanket was done; that baby was coming either way. I had agreed to be my neighbor's babysitter if she happened to go into labor, and if her mother hadn't arrived yet to watch her son. Her water had broken, and she was feeling anxious to get to the hospital that was at least a twenty-five-minute drive. I wrapped my oversized cardigan around me, slipped my flip flops on, and ran down the driveway in the dark. I felt so alive. Life was coming into the world, and I got to be a small, tiny part of it. The beauty of life is the ability to witness the joys and sorrows, life and death, and to support and help others through the process of both.

My mother just needed to hear it from me and my sisters that it was okay to have hospice start for my dad. She needed to hear that it didn't mean she was giving up on my dad, but she was doing what was best for him and, really, for her and all of us, too.

23

---◆─◆─◆---

The next month, on a weekend, I made a visit to my parents. They had a new caregiver starting and I wanted to do a meet and greet. I found my dad sitting in the side living room in his brown leather chair. I found him there many days now, either sleeping or watching something on his DVD player, or sitting quietly with a caregiver. A faint smile crossed his face. It was his way of saying hello to me now. If I got even a wisp of a smile, I took it as a good sign he recognized me, that he knew me. He didn't use my name and often wouldn't use any words when I arrived, but this worked for us now. I was happy. Simple pleasures. Little victories. "Hi, Dad! How's it going?" I smiled as big as I could. My dad was so innocent, gentle, and sweet. He didn't respond. If it was a good day, he might reply, "Where have you been?" I turned to the new caregiver and said, "Hi! I'm Drea, one of his daughters." I always made sure to point that out, to place myself immediately, so they didn't have to question if I was another caregiver, a different employee at the house, or anyone else. They usually replied with something like, "Oh, yes. I have heard about you." I often joked around with my dad and tried to carry a conversation with the caregiver while making sure Dad was also involved. So, after I said, "one of his daughters," I followed it with, "His favorite one," as a joke. I didn't truly believe that. Well, maybe once in a while I did. I turned to my dad and said, "Right, Dad? I'm your favorite?"

He looked at me and replied, dead serious, "You are *all* my favorite." A sentence. A meaningful multi-word sentence. And it was so purely sweet. I had to take a breath and push my tongue to the top of my mouth so I didn't cry. I let out a laugh instead.

Those moments were few and far between, but when they happened, it was like a little miracle. A splash of humor and hope to propel us forward. One day, my dad and I were eating lunch together. He normally ate in silence once his disease grew worse, often not looking up or at me directly. My mom commented he may not know me anymore. She may have been right. As we ate, I just watched him, searching his face for any recognition, anything that reminded me of Old Dad. Those were times I felt different with him. I felt as if the conversation could probably take any direction I wanted, and I probably had nothing to lose. I opened with, "Dad, this is pretty good, huh?" It was just his usual sandwich of ham and cheese on a sandwich flat, now cut into four, maybe even eight, pieces. Small enough so he didn't choke.

He didn't respond. I asked again. He said, "Yes."

Then I decided to go deeper. "Dad, you know you are my dad, right? That I am your daughter?"

He stopped eating. He looked up at me and, with hardly a smile but full of Old Dad charm, he responded loudly and clearly, "I hope so!" I may have even detected a hint of sarcasm, a well-shared family trait. I burst out laughing with a wave of relief and a little bit of surprise. My mother heard it from the other room. I repeated what my dad had just said, and she laughed too. My mother and I laughing together broke the constant feeling of hopelessness. *He knows me.* And if he doesn't know me, at least he *wants* to be my dad. Those were the moments that I truly believed he was aware of who I was to him. That maybe his communication wasn't the same, but that I was still important to him. That was enough for me, to get an answer and a response that made me laugh and feel that all wasn't lost. Another little victory.

Another evening, we sat around the table while Amy and Steve visited before summer got into full swing. My dad, after hours of silence that day, looked up and said, "We've been together a long time." He was right, and we all sat in silence and awe. My parents had been together for fifty years at that point. He was there, he knew, he remembered. I was then the speechless one. My heart was bursting for my mother and for us to witness my father speaking and for smiling while he did. The rest of dinner was quiet until he rubbed at his eyes. My mother hated when he did that. She said he would rub and then they would water and turn red and eventually need eye drops. He continued, and she began to get flustered. She shouted for someone to run to their room and get some eye drops. A tizzy broke out, and my sisters and I scrambled. I ran the way to their room, halfway across the house. I ran back to the table, and my dad sat with his eyes closed, as we all discussed the best way to give eye drops. Oh, the things my dad must have been thinking, listening to us cackle like hens, not a single one of us medically trained other than the man needing care himself. All of a sudden, his eyes popped open and for the second time that day, he spoke, "What the hell is going on?"

I burst out laughing. "Oh, my God, Dad. That should be the question of this crazy year, 2020," I said, laughing and agreeing with him. *What the hell was going on?*

And that's when Liza said what we often said when my dad did something that reminded us of who he used to be, "Oh, there's Old Dad!" and we all laughed, and the situation was diffused. My dad's eye was fine and so were we, as long as we could laugh and still see a glimpse of his humor and personality that we so missed.

24

It was a muggy, July day, and my parents' forty-seventh wedding anniversary. I wanted to make their day special—well, as special as it could be, so I planned to spend the afternoon and early evening with them. My mom and I both knew the celebration was more for her now. I knew this too, and, in an effort to lessen the blow, I didn't want her to be alone, even if she was with my dad. A part of the disease that is painful for loved ones is the idea that someone is gone before they are actually gone. My father's increasing difficulty with getting in and out of their bed was taking its toll on my mother physically, so she and the hospice nurse decided it was time for my dad to have a hospital bed. My parents' bedroom was large enough to accommodate both my parents' queen bed, as well as my dad's new, single hospital bed. When I saw it for the first time, I was somewhat horrified. I imagined a bed like I had at the hospital when I gave birth—large, white, with big arm rails on the side, and modern. Instead, my father had a small brown metal bed, with small metal bars that went up and down, if you forced them hard enough. After I saw the bed the first time, I texted my sisters, "Um… what is this bed? It looks like it belongs in a polio ward in the 1950s!"

My mom said, "I know. It doesn't look like much, but look what it can do!" and she showed me how it went up and down and higher and lower with the remote control attached to it. Then she said she would make the bed with some new pretty sheets, and it would look better and be cozier. My mother had that way. She could make any bed look fit for a king. Pillows and fine blankets and gorgeous patterns and textures were my mother's expertise. Her gift was her decorating skills. My dad had always said she had the vision, and he supplied the money and sometimes, the manpower. They were a team. On that day, they were still a team. My mother sat by his bedside then. He was in bed indefinitely due to a foot infection. If the caregiver wasn't there, my mother was at my dad's side, only leaving to use the restroom. She read to him or called a friend on the phone or watched a show on her iPad. Their bedroom had a door that led to a small deck, and beyond that was a beautiful manmade stream and garden. My father loved to look out at it and watch the clouds move and trees sway. My mother didn't leave his side that day. Much as in their life together, she never left his side. She was always his support, his travel companion, the voice he looked forward to hearing every night on his way home from work, and his partner in all things.

When they were first married, my father was finishing his last year of medical school, and my mother was working. She was bringing home their only income. She fully supported him then, and she fully supported him still in all his needs. My father was able to provide for them financially over the years, and my parents saved and prepared for the future. A future that might, unfortunately, turn out the way that it was—that someone would be dependent and need nursing and caregivers full-time, as my father did. My mother was to be admired for her commitment to my father. She was his voice now. His advocate. She spoke for him, stood up for him, and demanded he get the best of the best. She knew he deserved no less. She spent hours on the phone discussing his health care needs, sorting out health insurance, researching convalescence supplies he needed to continue living at home, finding caregivers to trust, and then more time training them and assisting them.

As my father grew more dependent, she hated leaving him alone, even with a caregiver. She was afraid something may happen in her absence. That he would need her or that for that brief time she went out, he would want her, and she wouldn't be there to comfort him. She even worried at times he would die while she was gone. I think she was getting swallowed by the role of caregiver and the guilt that comes along with finding time for herself, for doing the things she wanted to do that didn't involve being my dad's caregiver. She just wanted to be his wife, and now those lines were blurred. Her freedom was limited outside of the house, and her only role in life seemed to be to take care of my dad. I felt sad for her, but I also felt sad for *us*. She had joined a support group that "met" by phone once a week for caregivers and loved ones of those with dementia or Alzheimer's, but that was her only real time "away" lately. One day, she called me, and we finally discussed the elephant in the room. We discussed the usual stuff and then she finally admitted she missed me. She missed just being able to leave and come to visit and spend time with me, with her grandchildren. She regretted that when I visited, it was to help with Dad and not spend time talking with her or going out to lunch.

"Mom, I know. I know it's no one's fault Dad is sick, but it sucks. It sucks for him, for you, and for what I had hoped for us," I told her while trying to remain calm and sensitive to the situation. I had gone down to my basement to ensure I had some quiet and privacy away from my children when my mom called that day. I stared at the pipes that lined the ceiling and felt the cool cement on my feet while I paced as we talked.

"Andrea, I know. I wanted more for us, too. I wanted to be involved in my grandchildren's lives more. This is the time when Dad and I should be helping you, and instead, you are helping us. I miss my kids. I miss being able to be there for all of you," my mother said back just as calmly. We discussed more and both cried. I told her this situation was so complicated, and none of us knew how to completely do it the "right" way, but we could try and love each other and give each other grace in those times.

Air. Fresh air. Having this conversation with my mother was as if a huge weight had been lifted. I felt as if she had given me a huge hug over the phone. We could openly admit how unfair this was, and it felt so good to hear my mom say she missed me and that she agreed that this situation sucked. I know my thoughts were selfish at times, but sharing this with her was, I felt, my way of saying

I loved her and that I still needed her. I think as a mother, it was important for her to hear that she still had a role outside of being my dad's caregiver. That she was loved and supported and needed by others, even if she couldn't be all she wanted to be for us all. She was still a mother and grandmother and mother-in-law. We knew. We remembered.

I prepared dinner for my parents the evening of their anniversary and brought it to their room. Gone were the days of dining in fancy restaurants, first-class flights, and expensive jewelry given as gifts. My parents ate dinner in their bedroom on their anniversary. The room was adorned by beautiful wall hangings and mission style furniture, but now it took on the look of a private hospital room. My father had a table that could slide over his bed on wheels, endless supplies like chucks to keep his bed dry, boxes of latex gloves, and incontinence items. He wore a bandana around his neck to protect his clothing from any spills. My mother kept him well-groomed, hiring her hairstylist to come to the house and cut his hair and trim his nails. She thought of everything, and over the years as a doctor's wife, she had taken mental notes on how to care for wounds and other ailments. She was truly his guardian angel and nurse, and this was evident in the mass amount of medical supplies she kept stocked in closets throughout the house. I knew where I could get a bottle of peroxide, a box of gauze, or an extra toothbrush if the stores ever shut down.

I took a picture of my parents together. My dad attempted a smile. Dad wasn't gone; he was just different. I decided to get my parents wedding album and bring it to share with them. I opened it up and showed them the pictures. The white leather album had started to turn yellow with time, but it was still in excellent condition. We laughed about how much hair people had and how the color was drastically different. We laughed at the styles of the dresses, and my mother recalled how hot that day had been. I showed my dad a picture of my mom and said, "Wow. Isn't she beautiful?" He nodded his head in agreement. I asked my dad a few times who people were, to see if he could name anyone. He saw his own parents and said "father" about his dad. My mom and I looked at each other and smiled. I told my dad he was *my* father. I asked him if he knew that. No response. I then asked, "Do you want to be my dad?" and without hesitation he answered, "Yes!" *Well, then*, I thought, *that's good enough for me*. I knew I had to now phrase questions in the form that required only "yes" or "no" answers.

At the end, I closed the album, and my dad said, "Put it away safe." He didn't want it ruined, destroyed, or lost, I assumed. *Don't worry, Dad. I'll protect these memories.*

25

---◆—◆—◆---

The silence had begun to grow between my father and I during our visits, as his disease progressed. I sat at his side while he lay in bed, and unless I filled the room with my voice, there was quiet. Summer had once again slipped into a New England fall. It was too cold for the door or window to be open to listen to the stream outside, and there was no TV in my parents' room. My dad occasionally watched a movie on a DVD player, but it wasn't out that day. I looked at my phone and then it struck me. *Music.* My dad had grown up taking piano lessons and playing the black shiny grand piano in my grandparents' home. A piano that was a grandchild magnet. Every visit, we ran to it and banged away on the ivory keys, feeling like Mozart but probably sounding like some sort of warped musical circus. I never heard my father play piano, one wish I would have loved fulfilled in his retirement.

My father had encouraged me to take violin lessons when I expressed interest in the fourth grade. I remember running across the lawn with my rental violin in hand, as the case banged against my leg. It was an exciting time, but the newness wore off quickly, and violin was not the easiest instrument to learn. I asked to quit multiple times, but my father said no. He pushed me to continue through high school and to play with the high school orchestra. My first class I took for all four years of high school was orchestra, and it also was my only solid A I received in high school. My dad wouldn't let me give up, and looking back now, I am grateful for that. Our orchestra traveled to Europe twice in high school to play small concerts, and some of my closest friends were my fellow violinists and cellists.

My parents often went to the theater, and one of my dad's favorite musicals was *Jersey Boys*, which featured the music of Frankie Valli and the Four Seasons, a band from the 1960s. My dad operated on his unconscious patients to music, and often his residents made mixed tapes or CDs for him, and my dad was usually willing to try new things. Sometimes he expressed interest in the music my sisters and I listened to, so we would sneak a CD into his car for him or buy him one as a gift. That was often our connection. I knew that music was important for Alzheimer's patients. I knew that music can often stimulate memories, or a patient who lacks speech might remember how to sing a song. My father had no trouble hearing, as we often figured out when he shushed us to hear where my mother might be in the house, or he piped up hours after a conversation ended to ask us what we had been talking about. When my dad was hardly talking, we celebrated Jacob's birthday at my parents' house. We all sat around the dining room table and sang "Happy Birthday" to Jacob. Dad sat at the head of the table, and as we sang, I looked at him. To my surprise, he was singing along. Not every word, but he was singing. He remembered. His mouth moved, and he had a slight smile as he stared at Jacob and the birthday cake. Another moment to make me want to burst into tears. I was so happy Jacob had his grandfather singing to him.

So that day, to fill the silence, I turned on an app on my phone that played music and chose a station called "The 60s." I loved that station and knew my dad might recognize a lot of the music. The song we danced to at my wedding was "You are the Sunshine of My Life" by Stevie Wonder. I was hoping we would hear that song that day to see if it triggered a thought or memory for my dad. Instead, we listened to other music, and I looked at my father as I started the music and said, "Want to listen to some music with me?"

His eyes widened and he said, "Okay."

The music started to play and I smiled. "Do you know this one?"

A few seconds passed and then my dad said, "Yes." He seemed to lighten a bit. Relax a little. His face softened; his eyes seemed to get their twinkle back. We sat listening to the music. I nodded my head to the beat, once in a while glancing at him to see what he was doing. He had his eyes open. I wondered if the music had transported him back to another time. After a few songs, I decided to let my dad rest. I didn't want to overdo it, so I said goodbye and said, "Wasn't that fun?" He nodded yes. I could sense his mood was calmer, relaxed, and maybe even happy, from the subtlest smile across his face.

Another visit a few months later, I sat in the living room with my mother, and I heard my father and his caregiver listening to music in his room. It was pop music, loud and somewhat painful to listen to, even for me as someone thirty years younger than my dad. I got up, went in the room, and asked, "Dad, do you really like this music?" I didn't wait for an answer from either of them. I asked it more to imply I didn't like it on behalf of my dad. I knew it wasn't his choice, and the caregiver had just turned on the radio and left it, but instead, I searched for a classical station. I eventually found one that settled on some soothing orchestra piece and turned the volume down a bit. The caregiver agreed it sounded a bit nicer. My dad's face relaxed, and he drifted off to sleep a few minutes later. I knew my abilities with my father were limited at that point. A hand to be held, a shoulder to rub, a blanket to be tucked, but I could also adjust the music that entered his ears and enveloped his mind and body. It felt right and peaceful. My mother told me that, after that day, he continued to listen to classical music as he slept at night to keep him calm. When she told me, I felt as though I had contributed a little bit to his palliative care. I wasn't a clinician or a hired caregiver; I was just a daughter trying to make her dad comfortable. My heart felt full and happy that I could do something to help, as simple as it seemed. My life seemed to center around nurturing people, and I felt successful in that moment with my dad. I was proud I was able to help him, and I realized that my joy of classical music came from playing the violin for years, and my father was the driving force behind that. Our musical world had come full circle.

Music was truly a universal connection and always was an important part of carrying me through my father's illness. When I was happy, I turned on a dance tune and called my kids to the kitchen to have a dance party. When I needed to feel calm, I tuned in to the "spa music" station, closed my eyes, and took some deep breaths or took a shower listening to it. If I was alone in the car, I belted out a tune or cried in private. I partnered my walks for my physical and mental health with a favorite playlist. It was my release. It was my therapy. It was my way of transporting myself to another world or time, or a way to connect with my dad when we were together or even apart.

26

---◈—◈—◈---

As my father declined in his illness, his wardrobe vastly changed from handmade business suits to sweatpants, and finally, a hospital johnny. His transformation from academic surgeon to patient was complete. His copious number of business shirts, suits, and ties hadn't been worn in a few years, and even if he had a place to wear them, they didn't fit anymore due to his weight loss.

I was leaving after a visit one day, and my mom said, "Oh wait. I want you to take these. Just donate them," and she handed me three small clear plastic bins. They were stuffed full of all of my dad's ties. My father wore ties almost every day of his career. I took the bins and carried them out to my van. I placed them in the trunk, slowly, like they were delicate jewels. Those ties represented so much of my father. So many memories. I was sad to have another chapter close in his life but thought, *Well, maybe someone else can benefit from these in the working world.* The majority of them were either handmade or purchased from high-end places, so they were excellent quality that had stood the test of time. I brought the bins into my house and placed them in my hall closet, like a recently discovered hidden treasure that I wasn't ready to share with the world. I closed the doors and just wanted to keep them safe for a while. To keep them close to me. They were in my trusted hands, and there was no rush to donate them. I wasn't ready to let them go.

A few days later, I decided I could not bring myself to donate them. I had donated other clothes of my father's over time, but these felt more personal. I wanted to keep them for myself, at least for the time being. I had seen a lot of people make pillows or bears out of their loved ones' shirts, but I knew that wasn't for my family. My dad didn't have a shirt he wore that was significant to any of us. Then it hit me. I thought, *I bet there is something we can make with these ties.* I opened the bins and dumped them on my dining room table. With the ties came the smell of my dad's faint cologne, my parents' house, and some whiffs of my mother's scent as well. Had she kissed them goodbye? Had she held them close before packaging them away? I picked up a few and smelled them. *Oh, Dad.* I felt their cool silkiness on my skin. I rubbed my cheek with them, and it felt comforting, like a hug from my dad. I looked through the piles and recognized many of them from family events or pictures taken in his leadership capacity at work. I began to wonder about all of the ties and where they had been worn. Maybe one of these ties had been in the newspaper I had spotted my dad in years before one day on a lunch break. A coworker was sitting across from me, reading the newspaper, and as I bit into my sandwich, I looked up and saw my father's face. I focused closer on the paper in front of me and said, "Is that my dad?" I was living in New Hampshire, my father in Illinois, and there was his face, staring back at me on the back of a national newspaper. He was holding a bag of synthetic blood for a story relating to a study he was working on for traumatic injuries. My dad got a real kick out of that when I called him after work to tell him what I had seen, and so did I.

The wheels began to turn in my head, as I looked at the mountain of ties in front of me. I looked up tie pillows online. *This could work.* I started pulling out the ones I knew well, the ones I felt represented him best. The ones I remembered him wearing. I knew I had my own pictures to look at to place some of them in time, but I also knew I could reference the internet as well, as much of my dad's career was well-documented. Thank you to the gift of the internet. My plan was to make a pillow for my mother—rather, have a pillow made, as I did not inherit the natural or even trained ability to sew or use a sewing machine. I found a woman in California, during my internet search, who made beautiful pillows and contacted her, asking how to proceed. Time passed, and I never got to the post office to ship the ties out. It also didn't feel right anymore to release these ties to a stranger. I was becoming more attached to them the longer they sat in my closet. I realized I had to re-think my plan. I was protective of these materials, these memories. I wanted to honor them appropriately and make something new with them. I did not want to give them away or forget them. I knew it was time for the ties to be passed on, their original purpose having been served, but I felt they still had life in them. Something left to give back, a way to make them last forever.

My in-laws were coming to visit, and my mother-in-law was an extremely talented seamstress and quilter. *Why hadn't I considered this before?* When I asked her what she thought, she quickly responded, "Of course! Show me a picture, and we can do this." I had faith in her abilities as she had made quilts, blankets, pajamas for my children, my three sister-in-law's wedding dresses, and the baptismal gown for my three children, among many other items. Upon a trip to visit my in-laws, I finally remembered to bring the ties with me. I had over fifty ties. We dumped them all on *her* dining room table. My in-laws had been a support for me during my father's illness. They were some of the first people I told, outside of my immediate family. They were gentle, caring, and sorry for my family and the man they had gotten to know over sixteen years. I felt comforted and loved by them through the process. They had both survived cancer and an open-heart surgery, and their compassion was always there. My mother-in-law had lost her own mother at a young age, as a new mother with four small children, so she knew the pain and struggle to balance an ailing parent with being one herself. She said to me one day that she had wished she didn't feel as if she had to choose between her children and her mother back then, and I knew exactly what she meant. She said it was worth it for me to leave my children with Denis, so I could spend time with my dad whenever I needed or wanted to, and I realized she was right.

My mother-in-law eyed the ties splayed out on the table. Kids ran through the kitchen in a flurry of voices and footsteps. "Whoa! That's a lot of ties!" my son exclaimed. *No kidding,* I thought.

After realizing we had plenty of ties she said, "Why don't we make a pillow for you, too?"

I hadn't even thought of myself. When we realized we had even more ties, she suggested making some for my sisters as well. I was excited and felt full of love to give. I was going to be able to give my mother a piece of my father, as well as my sisters and I.

The irony was not lost on me as we cut the ties up, sewed them, and made something new. My father sewed for a living. He grafted skin from one part of the body and made something new from it. I felt as if we were our own version of surgeons, cutting and sewing. My mother-in-law was precise, methodical, and dedicated to her craft as well. As I handed her the ties, she said, "Oh, you are going to help me." I panicked. The sewing machine and I were not friends. She had tried to teach me years before, but I had forgotten and was overwhelmed by it all. She pulled out her second sewing machine and placed it on the table for me. I swallowed hard.

"I don't want to mess this up," I said with a panic and nervousness to my voice, trying to laugh.

"You can't. I will come help you when you need me

to. I'll be right over here working on some as well," she said with reassurance, a smile, and all the confidence in the world. She gave me a small task, and I got to work. I did screw up a few times, but she came to my side and rescued me. She helped me. She guided me. She knew how important this was to me, and her act of service was pure love and compassion. I felt as if she understood what this meant—to honor my dad, to help my mother, and to keep memories alive. She corrected her own work if she didn't feel it was perfect, while I watched and learned from her. She let me pick the fabric backing and the patterns from her piles and piles of extra cloth she kept in her "stash." Her work was my work, and we shared this process of collaboration and beauty. We saw that something had changed and was no longer the same but that it was still beautiful, useful, and memorable. These ties could still be loved and kept close to us. There was still a bit of what *was* in the something that now *is*. A glimmer of the past, mixed with different patterns and shapes. Memories are like that. They take on new shape or meaning over time. They can be carried on by the next generation, and they can be retold and given a new life. They can offer comfort, support, and a place to rest our weary heads. We can hold on, we can honor, and we can see the beauty and light in something we thought was gone. We can embrace what remains.

We can still learn and experience new things. We can bond with others over our losses and find a connection to keep going, to feel loved. Our support structure may not be what we had or who we had envisioned, but life is like that. It can surprise you with the beauty of the unexpected joy in a sea of darkness. It's like the day I got a message on Facebook from someone, asking me if Dr. Gamelli was my father. I verified he was and then began an exchange and a story of this woman's brother whom my father had saved thirty years prior. She was a child when it happened, but her mother had recently filled her in on the details, and she wanted to reach out to my father to share her gratitude and let him know how well her brother was doing. Her story was unexpected, but beautiful and special for my family to hear from her so many years later. It was what I needed that day, after spending the day before with my father and feeling pretty sure he had no idea of my identity as Andrea, or even his daughter. I could no longer depend on him to share his past with me, but there was this gift of stories from others that continued to teach me about my father, to weave together a past, to fill in the gaps, and to keep his memory alive through and for others.

When we finished the pillow, we showed my father-in-law. He walked over to the ironing board, quiet and calm, ever the gentleman. He was the hardworking, strong farmer with a heart of gold. He looked at the pillow and, with a tear in his eye, said, "Your mother is going to love this."

This gift, this process, and this memory we had created was what life was all about. Supporting each other, lifting each other up, showing love and strength, guidance, motivation, and confidence. Compassion. These were the ties that bound us, literally. Just as my relationship with my dad took a different direction, a new purpose, these ties had been given a new life, a new beauty, an unexpected joy. My mother-in-law helped my father's memory stay alive for my mother, sisters, and me. It was a merging of my family across both sides, a closing of a circle. When I gave my mother the pillow, she opened the gift bag, pulled it out gently, and stared at it. She quietly closed her eyes, fought back tears, and just hugged it close. "Oh, Andrea. It's beautiful. Thank you for this," she said while holding it.

I learned to use the sewing machine again. I may forget again, but I know I can ask for help from those who love me, to show the way, offer support, and remind me.

27

---◆◆◆---

My mother has told me the story of my birth many times over the years when I asked, when my birthday passed each year, or to bond over our shared journey of motherhood. My birthday came three weeks late on a hot August day. I was born within an hour of my mother first feeling labor pains and came out very sick with pneumonia. My first ten days was spent in the NICU until I was released to go home. Each time she shared this story with me, my mother added in more details. It wasn't until I was an adult that I learned how my father, being a new surgical attending at the same hospital, had come to hold me in the NICU every day at noon. As a parent now, I can't imagine how hard it was for my parents to see their sick baby struggling to survive. At my wedding, my father gave a toast referencing my birth and how, for my wedding ceremony, in sharp contrast to my birth, I was very "on time." The crowd chuckled. He then followed that statement with his own vulnerability and admitted for the first time I had ever heard that, as a surgeon, he felt very helpless following my birth and my fight to live. I will never remember my own birth and stay in the NICU, but knowing my father was there to comfort me will always remind me of his love from the very beginning.

***

My dad lay in his bed, looking out the windows down the backyard. His tie pillow sat to one side of him. The view of the mountains just beyond the closed windows and snow-covered hill was his view for the last few weeks. This time, he was bed bound for longer and not able to get out of bed. It marked the beginning of him never walking again. His foot was still not healed, and he didn't comment or seem to notice that he had been in bed for so long. As my mother had said from the beginning of his diagnosis, "He never complains."

I came to his bedside and gently said with a big smile, "Hi, Dad." His eyes shifted quickly from the windows to my face. A few seconds passed, and then there it was—a faint smile. At that point, I had been self-quarantining for a while with my kids, since it was Christmas break, so I didn't have to wear a mask to visit him. I had decided that his emotional and mental health, as well as mine, was more important than wearing a mask. He studied my face for a while. His eyes didn't leave me. The pandemic had been raging for nine months by that time, and my dad's Alzheimer's for four years, at least known to us. The outside world was slower. No one was really doing much of anything. Quick trips to the grocery store, a run into a restaurant for take-out, and maybe a walk around the block were still the extent of my life. My children were learning at home, and my husband still went to work but with social distancing and a mask. We had a few scares and had to test for COVID and quarantine for a week or so a few times.

I said to my dad after a little while, "Dad, it's a crazy world out there. You should be happy you retired. The medical field is insane right now." I felt like I was straight out of a science fiction movie with my recounting of the outside world. *I hope he knows what I said. Better yet, I hope he believed me.* As I said this, I realized how grateful I was that he was retired. The pandemic would surely have caused so much added stress to an already stressful profession. I would have always worried he would contract it or pass it along to my mother, if he was still in the hospital setting.

Overall and more so, I was grateful that in my father's current state in life, he wasn't actually missing much. Life wasn't really going on normally anywhere anymore. He spent his days in bed watching a movie, listening to music, or having a caregiver read to him. He underwent clothing changes, incontinence changes, dressing changes on his foot, and sponge baths. He welcomed a visit from a loved one and especially enjoyed my mother's bedside company. His life was slow, probably confusing, and most likely boring, and maybe even scary at times if he forgot or questioned why all the different people came and went in his room. Not too much unlike all of our lives, at some point. I was grateful he wasn't missing parties, the theater, traveling back to Illinois to visit friends, or attending other group events. Either way, Alzheimer's or not, it wouldn't have been safe or recommended at his age. The outside world had slowly shut down like a sleeping giant, just like my father. It was scary but peaceful; it was unknown, yet simple. It didn't require much effort anymore, and things like a view of the mountains or listening to music were enough for most people. Meeting our basic needs was our primary concern as a human race. Things like toilet paper and groceries were the sought-after commodities. We realized as a country that having these things was enough at times and that life didn't need to hurry on; it could wait or pause for a while.

My father had lived an exciting, exhilarating, adrenaline-pumping life. He had traveled to six of the seven continents and achieved a level of status only some doctors dream of for their careers. It was his time to rest. It was the world's time to rest—to rejuvenate and focus on the important things in life, like family and relationships. None of us were sure when life would resume its "normal" status. I knew my father would never resume the status he had before Alzheimer's, but I had accepted that fact. He wasn't missing out. He was doing what we all were. We were slowing down and looking forward to each other's company. A hug. A smile without a mask.

I pulled up my dad's blanket and said with a little laugh, "Want to go skiing today?" I wanted to see his reaction. It was blank. "Okay, maybe another day. It's really windy and cold."

I had recently skied with my daughter, and while she took a lesson, I did some runs alone. I rode the chairlift alone. I had never done that in my entire life. The pandemic, coupled with the fact my daughter was in a lesson, forced me to be alone, and as I sat on the chairlift, I breathed the cold air in and thought of my dad. I thought he probably had ridden chairlifts alone and that I could do it too. I knew he would be proud of me for doing it. If my father could ski at sixty-five, I could do it at forty-one. I felt invigorated by his spirit that day. I teared up thinking of us being together, skiing as we had in the past. I had no one to talk to on the chairlift, but my thoughts of my father were my companion. He now lay in a bed, only looking at mountains, not skiing on them. He had lived, he had enjoyed his life, he had taken risks, and I am sure had blind faith at times in his career. It was my turn to have the same, trust myself, and believe in myself. I was inspired, comforted, and strong. Thank you, Dad.

Acknowledgments

I would like to express my sincere appreciation to all of those who supported me in the writing of this memoir. First and foremost, my gratitude to my mother for her constant encouragement, patience, willingness to listen, and discuss our life and my father's disease openly with me. I thank her for allowing me to share our family's story and my father's story, in an honest and vulnerable way. I want to honor my father and thank him for providing me the ability to believe in myself and achieve my goals and also as the inspiration and love behind this memoir. His legacy is alive and well. I thank my sisters for being my cheerleaders and confidants while letting me share intimate moments in all of our lives. I appreciate my children for understanding that sometimes Mom needed to be alone to focus and for being excited as I finished the book and asked often for an "autographed copy". My heartfelt thanks to my extended family and friends for supporting me along my journey and for often being a special part of it. I also want to thank Danielle Anderson, my editor, for giving me the push I needed to continue writing, sharing, and "diving deep" into my emotions and memories to craft my best book possible. I want to thank Jade Rawlings for my beautiful cover design and her patience with me throughout the process. And lastly, but never least, I want to thank my husband, Denis, for always supporting my need for quiet and space while I wrote. His love and encouragement kept me going. He listened to every page I wrote as I read it aloud to him and provided honest feedback. He brainstormed book titles with me, printed my manuscript numerous times so I could edit, shared with me in my grief, and reminded me of my strength. To all the memoirists that share their story and encourage others to do the same, I am grateful for their inspiration and guidance along this powerful journey of healing and sharing.

About the Author

This is Andrea Couture's first memoir and book. She has a Bachelor of Arts degree in Journalism from Saint Michael's College in Vermont. Andrea is passionate about sharing her story and experience and supporting others in the Alzheimer's community and the world. She lives in New Hampshire with her husband, three children, and her dog.

Made in the USA
Monee, IL
01 October 2022

15030290R00129